FREEDOM FROM BACK PAIN

FREEDOM FROM BACK PAIN

An Orthopedist's Self-Help Guide

Edward A. Abraham, M.D.

 Rodale Press   Emmaus, Pennsylvania

Printed in the United States of America on recycled paper, containing a high percentage of de-inked fiber.

Book design by Acey Lee
Figure illustrations by Susan Rosenberger
Medical illustrations by Ira Alan Grunther

Library of Congress Cataloging-in-Publication Data

Abraham, Edward A.
    Freedom from back pain.

    Includes index.
    1. Backache—Popular works. I. Title.
[DNLM: 1. Backache—prevention & control—popular works. WE 720 A159f]
RD768.A27   1986   617'.56   86–13095
ISBN   0–87857–657–6   hardcover
ISBN   0–87857–658–4   paperback

2 4 6 8 10 9 7 5 3 1   hardcover
2 4 6 8 10 9 7 5 3 1   paperback

Notice

This book is intended as a reference volume only, not as a medical manual or guide to self-treatment. If you suspect that you have a medical problem, you should seek competent medical help. The information here is intended to help you make informed decisions about your health.

To my friend Morty Stein, who touched the hearts of those who knew him in so many ways. His zest for life in spite of almost insurmountable physical limitations was a symbol to us all. Morty is no longer with us, but his spirit lives on in all those who try just a little harder each day. We all deeply miss him.

Contents

Acknowledgments

I would like to express my special appreciation to all the patients who made this book possible. Without countless hours of firsthand clinical experience, I would not have gained the insight to understand the range and depth of the problems faced by the back sufferer.

I thank my parents, Sam and Dora Abraham, for instilling in me an unshakeable sense of self-worth and the confidence to believe in my ability to achieve any goal. Since my father's death, my stepfather Bernie Golden has continued with encouragement.

To my children, Susie, Gary, Scott and Kelly, who have done without my presence for many days and nights while I pursued my career, I extend my deep love and affection.

I have the great fortune to be the nephew of a physician, Jack Zuckner, and his wife Phyllis, who in my formative years of schooling, guided and helped me in many ways. If not for them, my career would certainly have taken another direction.

I extend my appreciation to my associates and colleagues in evaluating the therapy clinic, especially to Marty Migdall, Larry Leifer and all the therapists and aides who helped to create a new concept in back care; to Vert Mooney, M.D., Bill McMaster, M.D., Michael Einbund, M.D., Jacob Rabinovich, M.D., and James Moore, M.D., who offered invaluable assistance; and to Sanford Anzel, M.D., and Theodore Waugh, M.D., who were the backbone of my early training in orthopedics.

Many thanks also to Coral Hoffman, Tony Midnight, Dan Whiteside and Jerry Holderman for their vital contributions in helping to formulate this book; to Murray Fisher for his invaluable aid in editing it; to Nancy Ingall, my secretary and right arm for 11 years, for her help in preparing the manuscript for publication; to the rest of my office staff who were there supporting me; and to Annie Barnes, who helped promote and present the manuscript for publication.

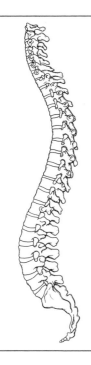

Don't Be a Victim of Pain

CHAPTER 1

Janet, in her mid-30's and a divorced mother of two teenage girls, managed her home while working as an escrow officer in a savings and loan. Though she loved her job, she hated sitting behind a desk all day, and the daily 45-minute commute in rush hour traffic frazzled her nerves.

At home there was a different kind of work. Janet's daughters were thoughtless and unconcerned about anything unrelated to the telephone or boys; they left the cooking, housework and laundry to Janet, which she rationalized as being okay—after all, it was the only exercise she got.

Janet's recent divorce had been an emotional bloodbath. A year earlier, her husband had left her for another woman. Following the final decree, she resolved to make herself over and went on a number of crash diets. She peeled off the pounds, but the heartache remained. Still, Janet did her best, trying hard to look, act and think younger than her years. Rarely asleep before midnight, she lived life to the fullest, no matter how empty it all seemed at the core.

Her salary was adequate, but the house was big, and hiring a gardener for yard work took financial priority over paying anyone to do odd jobs inside. Besides, she thought it was fun to putter around the house on weekends.

1

How Trouble Begins

One Saturday morning, Janet and one of her daughters started redecorating the girl's bedroom. By early afternoon, they'd almost finished hanging the new wallpaper. On a ladder, Janet bent to take the last sheet of pasted paper from her daughter's hands. It was a moment she would never forget.

Inexplicable pain seared down her back. She couldn't straighten up. Paralyzed with fear, she clutched the ladder until her daughter coaxed her down to the floor, where she lay for half an hour before the torment began to subside. It hadn't disappeared, of course, but only one wallpaper panel remained to hang. Never a quitter, Janet resolved to complete the job and staggered back up the ladder. By the time she'd finished the panel, the pain was back—and worse than before. Lightning stabs knifed down her left leg, red-hot and prickly. She had just suffered an acute attack of back pain.

Leaving the children to feed themselves, she managed to climb into bed. Every movement brought agony; there was no comfortable position. Sleep defied her. Eventually she gave up and dragged herself to the floor, a remedy for back pain that she'd heard others discuss. It didn't help, but she couldn't muster the courage to move again.

The next morning, her daughters found her. Together, the girls lifted her into bed. That afternoon, a neighbor persuaded Janet to go to a nearby hospital emergency room. Since her medical insurance policy covered such a visit, Janet agreed. Dressing, climbing into the car and out of it again was sheer agony. So was the two-hour wait before a doctor could see her.

Dazed with pain, she barely heard his advice: a week of complete bedrest, eased by muscle relaxants and pain killers. And she was to keep as still as possible at all times. Janet tried to explain that she couldn't afford bedrest. She had a job, income to earn, a home to run, children to take care of. A week in bed was unthinkable. Surely just being careful would be enough—that and the drugs prescribed. Again the doctor warned her, but Janet knew best. Pain killers would turn the trick. They'd have to.

They didn't.

After another sleepless night, Janet forced herself out of bed and managed to take a shower. The warm water relaxed her enough to provide a glimmer of hope. That glimmer faded, however, during her 45-minute commute to work. Driving seemed to make the pain stab with ever greater frequency.

Knowing she wouldn't last the whole day, Janet made the necessary arrangements. As soon as her escrows were in order, she went home. The drive was pure hell. Once again in bed, she called her neighbor to borrow a supply of sleeping pills.

For the first time in 48 hours, Janet slept.

Tuesday morning, she dragged herself to the family doctor. Pain prohibited a thorough examination, but he'd been her physician for years and knew she had no previous history of back problems. Palpating on and around her spine, the doctor found muscle spasm that severely limited her range of motion. Her reflexes were normal, yet she couldn't complete a sciatic nerve stretch-test. Pain flared down her leg; she had to stop.

The doctor's advice seemed as vague as her pain was real: bedrest, at least a week to start, either in the hospital or at home. Janet chose her home, but her idea of bedrest differed drastically from his. She was constantly in and out of bed, cooking meals, packing lunches and "tidying up" after the girls. On top of worrying about her inability to move without pain, she fretted about things at work, making dozens of calls to the office to stay in touch with various projects.

At the end of the week, Janet begged her doctor to allow her to return to work. Aware of her situation, he reluctantly agreed. Armed with prescription drugs, Janet returned to the savings and loan.

Choosing to ignore her condition was her first mistake. Relying on medication was her second. Business as usual became the order of the day, but so did pain.

The children, of course, were glad to see Mom back in the swing of things. But as is far too often the case, her nearest and dearest stopped thinking about her needs and focused back on their own, adding to Janet's continuing stress. Still, it was her "obligation as a mother" and she stifled her resentment. Janet's social life, meanwhile, became nonexistent. By the time dinner was done and the dishes were washed, she had little or no desire to do anything but wash down a Valium with brandy and collapse into bed.

At work she forced a smile, having decided to grin and bear it. That smile didn't last. Two weeks after going back, the grueling commute and what she considered her co-workers' lack of compassion began to pall. In the third week, she found herself snapping at them, always feeling irritable and angry. Pain made it difficult to think. Finally, she began calling in sick. Absenteeism became easier to consider in the face of anguish.

Beyond pills and bedrest, she knew of no other recourse than alcohol to assuage the agony. Cocktail hour started earlier every day. Her diet became a thing of the past. So did her belief that medication could handle pain.

Six weeks after she'd first seen him, Janet returned to the family doctor and agreed to hospitalization and a complete battery of tests. They were inconclusive. When her doctor reported this, Janet became hysterical and dissolved into tears. There *had* to be something truly wrong! She wasn't *faking* what she felt! There had to be an answer, some medical solution. What about surgery?

Wisely, her doctor explained that an operation would be a risk since there was no clear diagnosis of a surgical problem. Instead, he asked Janet to remain in the hospital—this time in traction—to guarantee complete immobility and total rest. Her health insurance would pay for such treatment and her mother volunteered to look after the children, so Janet agreed.

Traction was an ordeal. Even so, in just a few days, she noticed the pain had subsided slightly. That brought hope and she remained as still as possible (which, in traction, is *very* still). Her two weeks of immobility and cooperation paid off. Almost miraculously, the pain went away. Janet was certain she was cured.

Upon discharge from the hospital, her doctor prescribed an exercise program and encouraged her to investigate a local health spa specializing in back conditioning. Enthusiastically, she did as he suggested. Unfortunately, her insurance didn't cover such therapy, and the spa proved too expensive for her budget. No problem, Janet rationalized. She could always do the same exercises alone at home.

At first, things went beautifully. Janet's mother had set the house and kids back in order. There was a renewed atmosphere of cooperation and concern. Following doctor's orders, Janet did her exercises, was careful about lifting heavy objects, and slept flat on her back with a pillow tucked under her knees.

Three weeks later, she felt so good that she discontinued her routine. A new man had come into her life. Bob was outgoing and loved to dance. Surely, two nights a week at the disco made up for any silly regimen of boring, repetitious exercise. Work at the savings and loan was fun again. She went on another crash diet and lost 10 pounds. Best of all, she found emotional healing in making love, forgetting the hurts she'd harbored since her divorce. In fact, Bob became the new focus of her life.

Two months went by so smoothly and happily that she was totally unprepared for what was to happen. One morning, as she pulled into the parking lot at work, Janet couldn't get out of her car. In fact, she couldn't walk. Searing pain encompassed her, flashing down both legs, burning like flame.

This time her doctor couldn't even find a muscle spasm. In fact, he found no specific condition for which effective treatment might be prescribed. Desperate, Janet decided she needed another opinion and started "shopping doctors"—orthopedic specialists, chiropractors, acupuncturists, anyone who offered hope. She saw them all. But each brought disappointment and each represented another month or more in continued pain. Finally, when one doctor suggested to Janet that she might explore psychological counseling, she became hysterical and demanded surgery. It was her *back*, not her *mind*, that was causing her such anguish!

The Problem with Janet

When I first saw Janet, nearly three years had passed since her initial flare-up. There had been two operations including a second to correct a problem with the first. During that second surgery, two vertebrae had been fused. Neither procedure had relieved her pain.

Her mother pushed Janet's wheelchair into my office.

I don't think I've ever seen so much paraphernalia outside of an Intensive Care Unit. A neck brace was stuffed in a huge shoulder bag, which also held assorted medications. She had a special device attached to the wheelchair that held crutches, as well as a variety of canes for her to use, depending on how much pain she was suffering. Only partially ambulatory, she had to remove a back brace in order to be examined.

Unkempt and approaching obesity, Janet barely resembled the photograph she showed me, taken before her first seizure. And tragically, her life had deteriorated as much as her appearance. Total preoccupation with pain had turned her into a shrew; her children spent as much time as possible out of range of her sharp tongue. When they came home from school, she was often anxious and depressed, eager to lecture them on how her pain obligated them to take care of her. They lived on welfare, food stamps and what her mother could spare from her own meager Social Security checks. While she spoke wistfully about the possibility of returning to work, her expression told me she had other priorities. There were advantages, after all, to her immediate situation. Medical insurance policies had been consumed by the costs of her second operation, but the government could afford to pay her bills.

Pain was all she talked about—that, and what pain made it impossible for her to do. She couldn't bathe herself, or even go to the bathroom without assistance, and she left home only to seek more medical advice. She never allowed herself anything as frivolous as a social evening with friends, especially in light of the pain such effort might cause.

Janet's romance with Bob had gone the way of all her other relationships. At first, fearing she might lose him, she continued sleeping with him in spite of the pain. But pain and fear of more pain made her a dismal partner. Bob eventually moved on to greener pastures, explaining that he felt sadistic when they had sex.

She was still after relief from pain, but not, it seemed, if that meant she had to *do* anything to stop it. As her doctor, it was up to me to save her. Not that she was very optimistic; after all, numerous medical practitioners had failed her, just as her back had betrayed her. But she was still doctor shopping, and guess what she wanted: a third operation!

I didn't agree to that request. The effects of the two surgeries she'd already undergone had left her partially crippled, and it's likely she'll have to live with that for the rest of her life. So it was futile to talk of full recovery. At best, her improvement would be slight. But I offered what hope I could. A prescribed therapy program could extend her level of activity. A changed mental attitude could enhance her life. Possibly with time, regular exercise and motivation, Janet would see enough progress to make effort a reward in itself. Gently, I encouraged her to consider a regular program of physical therapy as the first step.

She looked away, tears in her eyes. "My pain won't let me," she cried. "I can't follow any kind of therapy program. It hurts too much. Besides, I tried that kind of thing way back at the beginning. It didn't work then, it won't work now."

The fatalism in her voice was like a knell, tolling defeat. Janet was in mourning for her life. For her, it was over. She had lost the battle for recovery. More accurately, she had surrendered to the pain.

I wish I could tell you there's a happy ending to Janet's story, but Janet is a back *loser*. Millions all over the world have stories that echo hers. Overwhelmed by anguish, they take what seems to be the easiest course, that of dependence—dependence on drugs, dependence on welfare, dependence on doctors, on anything except the one source that could bring at least some measure of freedom. Themselves.

You Are Not Alone

It doesn't have to be like that—not for Janet, not for anyone. But it is. In the United States alone, more than 70 million people are suffering from back problems. Five million of them are partially disabled. Another 6 million will develop back problems during the next year. Eighty percent of all

Americans will complain of spinal trouble before the age of 50, and after that age, you can count your blessings if chronic back pain isn't one of your major health concerns.

In fact, chances are that you're reading this book because you or someone you love suffers an acute or chronic back condition. At one time or another, just about everybody does. Whether you're young, old, male, female, white, black, red, yellow or brown, it's almost inevitable.

It's not surprising that we Americans spend 5 *billion dollars a year* for back examinations, treatment and therapy, not to mention the untold billions spent in disability claims, legal actions, lawsuit awards—and the fact that back pain is the single most significant factor in lost time on the job. No other affliction even comes close.

What's worse, with this overwhelming burden of suffering multiplied worldwide, next to nothing is being done to study the causes and cures for back problems. According to Alf Nachomson, M.D., of Sweden's Gotenburg University, an international authority on the subject, only 500 physicians throughout the world are trying to evaluate treatment of back pain, and no more than 50 scientists are working to discover the causes of what he calls "the world's most expensive health problem."

Janet's tragedy is legion and, sadly, it's being duplicated daily by millions who don't realize that surgery, even with all its modern improvements, cannot help 90 percent of back conditions.

Approximately 200,000 back surgeries will be performed this year in the United States alone; of these, 85 percent will be successful to a significant degree. Even so, a third of all back operations are followed by a second surgery. And what about the 15 percent that prove unsuccessful? That's 30,000 people who endured the anguish of back surgery only to find no relief from their pain—or to find that their pain had worsened.

Adding to this burden, until recently, has been the lack of any constructive outpatient program that could aid recovery. Prior to the last decade, once a back patient was discharged from a hospital, the only medical advice was "medication, light exercise and time." Most physicians, realizing there was little more they could do, washed their hands of the problem.

I wasn't content to overlook such massive suffering. That's why in 1973 I created Postural Therapeutics in Santa Ana, California, this country's first outpatient back rehabilitation clinic. Our treatment is a simple one: conservative therapy, aggressively applied.

Modern medicine today acknowledges that with back sufferers, pain is not the only problem and surgery is not the only answer. Through education, motivation and supervised exercise, patients *can* improve regardless of their current condition. What's more, they may get better faster than they thought they could.

At Postural Therapeutics, for example, using aggressive, conservative therapy, up to 70 percent of those enrolling in our group recovery programs return to work and an active social life within several months. Many will need to continue supervised therapy for a much longer period. Some may need a lifelong program to maintain freedom from physical limitation or as a safeguard against another painful episode. But that's a small price to pay, especially when one realizes the alternative is increasing immobility.

I'm sorry to say that we haven't been able to help everybody, but no therapeutic program will ever be entirely successful. Like Janet, our back losers have chosen to believe that pain is their only problem. Fixated on that belief, pain consumes their consciousness, destroying any other option. That's why we stress that pain is only a condition—a "given"—and that the behavior *caused* by pain is the real problem.

As with Janet, prolonged physical agony often results in profound psychological changes. Chronic sufferers undergo a personality adaptation of which they may not be fully aware. It's called Pain Behavior, and it can be even more destructive than the physical agony that prompts it. Until both the physical and psychological ramifications of pain are acknowledged and addressed, recovery remains a distant dream.

If any part of Janet's case history strikes a familiar nerve, you may be at a crossroads. The implications are tremendous; they could affect every aspect of your life. And no matter how much you want instant remission, no such cure exists. All doctors can do is offer guidance. It's your pain, your body, your life. Only you have the power to recover. And you *can* recover—if not completely, at least to a meaningful degree.

This book is a blueprint for that recovery. It's also a valuable resource on how to prevent the agony of an acute attack as well as how to relieve a chronic condition. If you're currently in the throes of either trauma, I want to help you understand your potential for improvement—not only physically, but in each pain-shattered area of any relationship, personal or professional. It's vital that you realize every way in which back pain can affect your life.

With a problem as complex as the cause and correction of back pain, this book may not be a panacea, but you'll find it's no placebo either. Read it with an open mind and take the advice I offer.

It can help. It could even change your life.

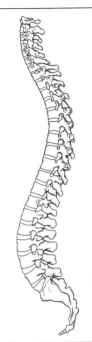

How Your Back Is Structured— And What Can Go Wrong

CHAPTER 2

gnorance lies at the root of fear. If you know how your body is structured and how it functions, it's easy to work with that body if anything goes wrong. Medical science knows one cardinal rule: Given half a chance, the body will heal itself. Ignorance of body basics denies us that half-chance, focusing us on fear instead of on recovery.

I've found that the average person knows more about what goes on under the hood of a car than about the most basic functions of the human body, and since you (not your doctor) are ultimately responsible for the maintenance of your body, it's important to acquire an elementary working knowledge of that body's basic equipment—in this case, the spine, the spinal cord and the muscles that affect your back's well-being.

Anatomy of the Spine

If you're confused by scientific facts, and many are, relax. I'll make this easy for you by sticking to basics. The spine is a long series of connecting bones. These bones are called vertebrae. Each one has a hollow portion designed to protect the cord of nerves leading downward from the brain.

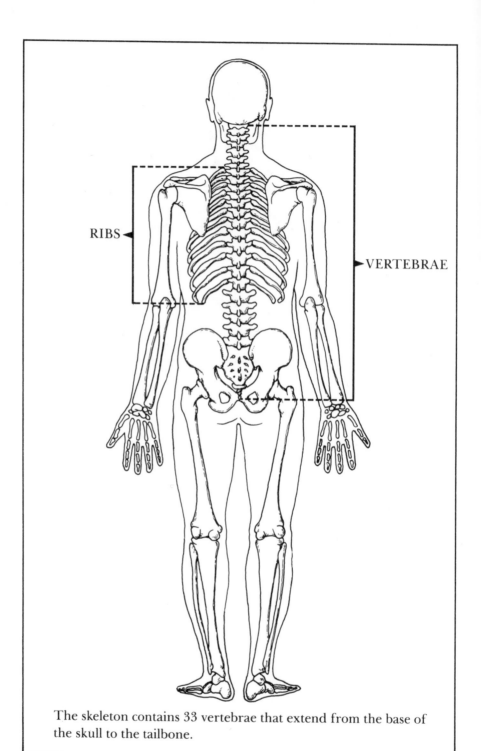

RIBS

VERTEBRAE

The skeleton contains 33 vertebrae that extend from the base of the skull to the tailbone.

Let's take a closer look at this structure, narrowing our focus to the individual vertebrae. Each is held in place by an intricate support system of muscle sheathing and ligaments, and each is separated from the other by a delicate, spongy pad which operates as a kind of shock absorber. This spongy pad is called a disc. Discs keep the vertebrae from abrading one another and make spinal motion possible with a minimum of adjustment.

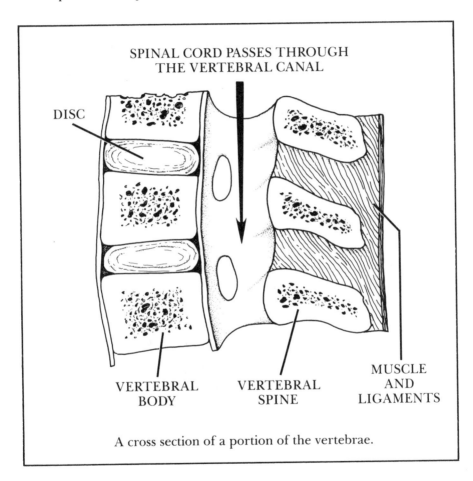

SPINAL CORD PASSES THROUGH
THE VERTEBRAL CANAL

DISC

MUSCLE
AND
LIGAMENTS

VERTEBRAL
BODY

VERTEBRAL
SPINE

A cross section of a portion of the vertebrae.

Your spine has five sections, the first three of which are most important for understanding how the back functions:

The *cervical* vertebrae link downward from the skull to the shoulders and become progressively larger as they descend. "Cervical" comes from the Latin word for neck. There are seven cervical vertebrae.

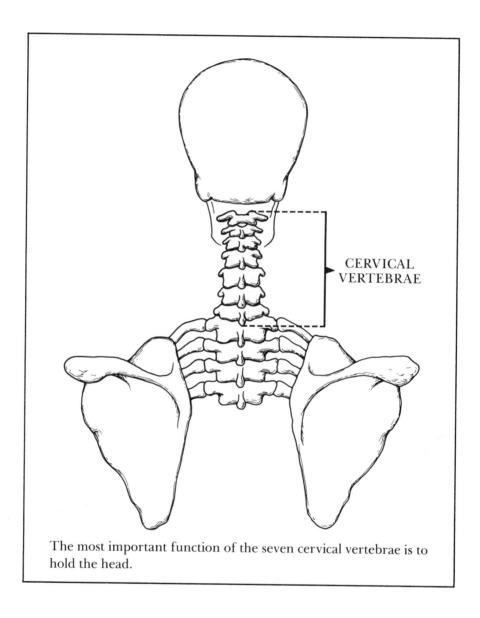

The most important function of the seven cervical vertebrae is to hold the head.

The *thoracic* portion of the spine runs downward from the cervical vertebrae, from the shoulders to the end of the rib cage. The thorax is that part of the body's trunk which is enclosed by the ribs. There are 12 thoracic vertebrae, just as there are 12 ribs.

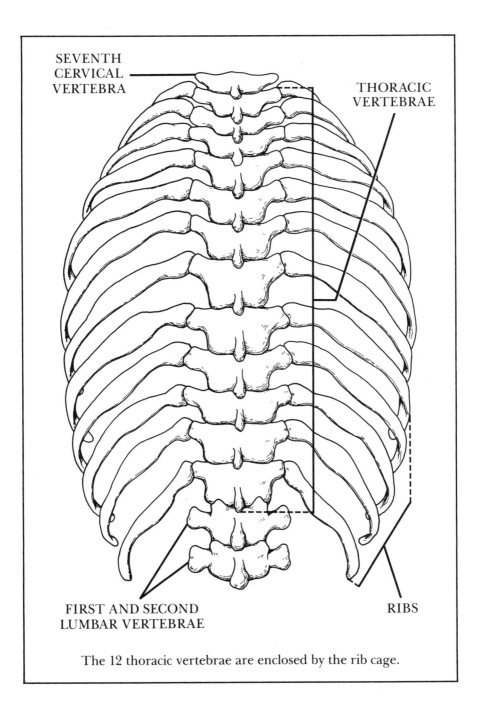

SEVENTH
CERVICAL
VERTEBRA

THORACIC
VERTEBRAE

FIRST AND SECOND
LUMBAR VERTEBRAE

RIBS

The 12 thoracic vertebrae are enclosed by the rib cage.

The *lumbar* vertebrae continue from below the ribs to the hips. Lumbar means "of or pertaining to the loins." These are the spine's heftiest vertebrae and there are five of them.

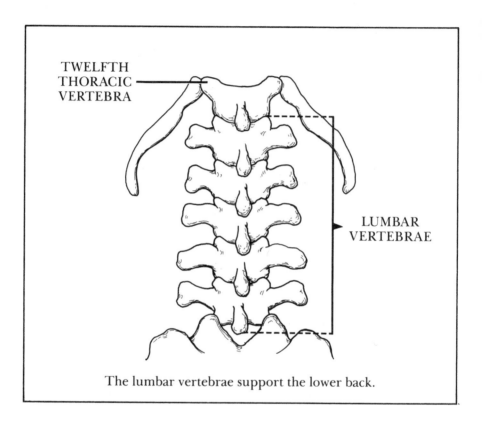

TWELFTH
THORACIC
VERTEBRA

LUMBAR
VERTEBRAE

The lumbar vertebrae support the lower back.

The remaining sections of the spine include the sacrum and the coccyx. The word "sacrum" comes from the Latin root word for "sacred" because this series of fused vertebrae was examined in sacrificial animals as a sign of a good or bad omen. "Coccyx" literally means "cuckoo" because the ancients thought this part of the spine resembled that bird's bill.

The five *sacral* vertebrae are fused to form a single triangular boneplate which curves inward at the base of the spine—roughly speaking, between the upper portion of the buttocks.

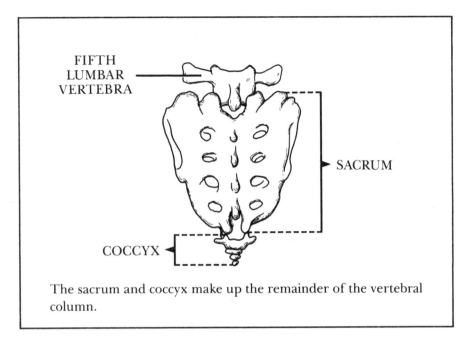

FIFTH
LUMBAR
VERTEBRA

SACRUM

COCCYX

The sacrum and coccyx make up the remainder of the vertebral column.

The four tiny *coccygeal* bones complete the spinal skeleton. The coccyx constitutes a tail-like appendage, presumably a vestigial "tail" inherited from our simian predecessors.

The spinal column provides us with three services. It supports the head and permits the torso to bend, turn, twist, etc. It also protects the spinal cord, that bundle of nerve fibers which connects the brain and the body.

Nerve impulses from the brain flow down the spine and out into the body through the spinal cord. Via the same path, impulses and sensations from within the body are telegraphed upward to the brain.

Nerves exit the spine through special openings, and each section of the spine protects the exit of specific nerve groupings. The cervical vertebrae, for example, shelter exits for nerves governing motions of the arms and hands. Thoracic vertebrae provide exits for nerves that direct activity within the torso and rib cage. Lumbar vertebrae house the exits for nerves having to do with motion of the lower limbs. Even the sacrum and coccyx deliver nerve pathways into the body.

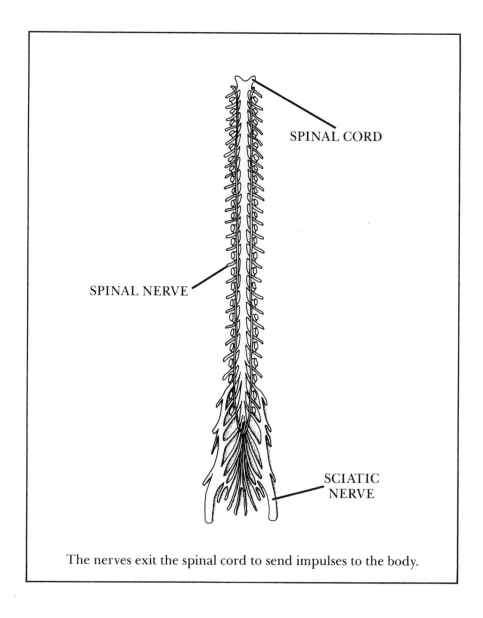

SPINAL CORD

SPINAL NERVE

SCIATIC NERVE

The nerves exit the spinal cord to send impulses to the body.

Let's take a closer look at the intimate juxtaposition of the vertebrae, the discs that cushion and separate them and the pathway of exiting nerves. Let's examine the lower lumbar area where the sciatic nerve leaves the spinal cord and extends downward through the legs.

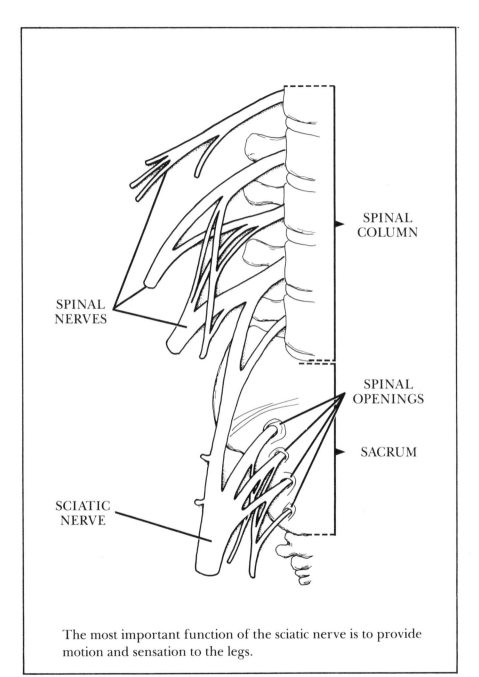

The most important function of the sciatic nerve is to provide motion and sensation to the legs.

Within the spinal cord itself are key ganglia (nerve centers) that process input from the body and "decide" whether to relay that input to the brain. These nerve relay centers are composed of the same gray matter as that within the brain itself. Each of the spine's basic sections has such relay centers and each is programmed to handle many decisions for us on a deep, subconscious level.

Once we've learned to walk, for example, we no longer have to consciously choose to put one foot in front of the other in order to perform that motion. Repetition has made this an automatic, programmed "choice" within the lumbar region's nerve relay center. Arm movements, such as automatic recoil (pulling your hand back from an open flame), are handled by a nerve relay center in the cervical area.

Thus, through the spinal cord, every thought formed in the brain is translated into action by the body and everything that happens in the body can be relayed back up to the brain. Since we're used to this happening as a matter of course, we may overlook the wonder of its complex simplicity. And yet, without a spinal *column*, we wouldn't be able to stand erect. Without a spinal *cord*, we wouldn't even be alive. Our very function as human beings depends upon these two elements, and they depend upon our masculature for flexibility, stability and support.

The Spine's Muscular Support System

There are specific muscles which stabilize and sheath the spinal column per se, primarily the sacrospinalis group that extends along the spine from the sacrum and hip bones to the base of the skull, the shorter of its fibers going from one vertebrae to the next, the longer fibers extending the whole length of the back.

Many of the body's other major muscle groups interact directly with the sacrospinalis to permit motions such as bending, lifting, lying down, getting up, reaching, twisting, walking, sitting, even sneezing. The psoas (pronounced "so-az"), for example, which has much to do with leg motions, has its points of origin along the spine from the level of the last rib downward, including all the lumbar vertebrae, and connects with muscles inside the upper part of the thigh.

The gluteal muscle groups (buttocks) also have an interrelation to the spinal support system. Their points of origin include the sacrum, and these

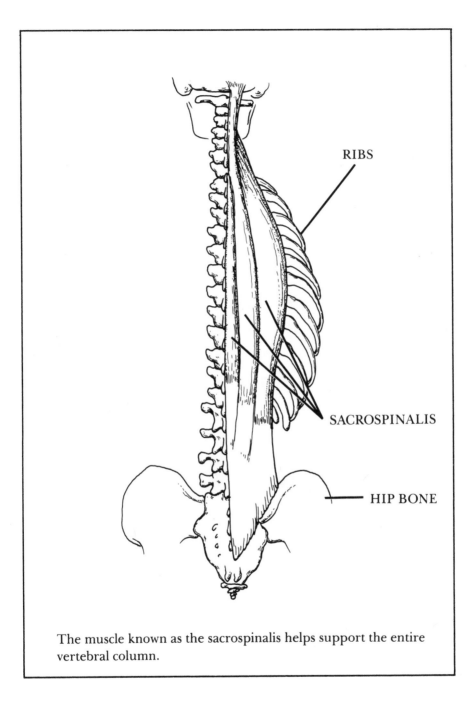

The muscle known as the sacrospinalis helps support the entire vertebral column.

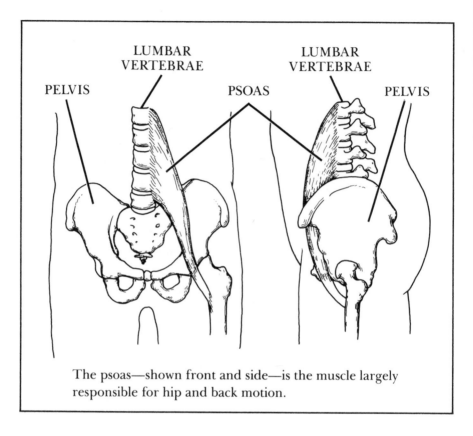

The psoas—shown front and side—is the muscle largely responsible for hip and back motion.

muscles are also important in moving lower limbs. Note the close connection with the sacrospinalis.

Any significant motion affects the spine's support system. The trapezius and upper trapezius groups—which have to do with moving the back, shoulders and head—originate along the spine from the level of the last rib to the base of the skull.

This intimate interaction between the spine and back muscles is what enables us to function with such a oneness of mind and body. The spinal cord carries a command from the brain. Within the spine, nerve relay centers process programmed performance and activate impulses that exit the spine to contract or release the appropriate muscle groups that move the body. At the same time, every other muscle group throughout the body adjusts to keep us in balance, constantly adapting automatically to the needs of whatever activity we're involved in.

What's more, our bodies handle muscular stress and strain as a matter of course. Well-balanced muscles in the upper torso, for instance, can reduce stress on the spine by approximately 30 percent. Well-toned abdominal muscles can reduce spinal stress by 50 percent. With such automatic balance, the spine remains free of the stress caused by focused pressure.

Did you know that simply standing erect focuses approximately one hundred pounds of pressure on the lumbar area of the spine? Lifting puts even more pressure on the lower spine. And yet even under extreme physical stress, the brain and body make the automatic adjustments to keep us moving toward what we want to accomplish—as long as the spine and muscles are synchronized and the muscles are balanced and well toned. Delicate, complex, with every function intricately related to the body's muscular

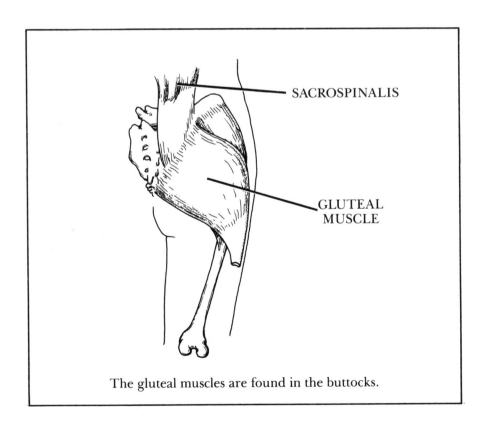

The gluteal muscles are found in the buttocks.

activity, the spine is a wonder of construction and capability. Designed to last a lifetime without problems, the spine and spinal cord provide us with the physical wherewithal to do, be and have whatever we desire.

What Can Go Wrong

Of course, the spine can be traumatized by physical injury, but specific injuries—such as fractures—constitute only a small percent of the causes for back suffering. In fact, that percentage is so small that I'm going to concentrate on what goes wrong in the vast majority of back conditions: The problem is usually associated with long-term habit patterns that induce

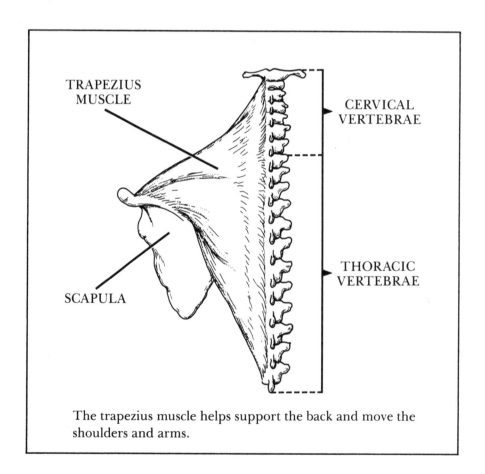

The trapezius muscle helps support the back and move the shoulders and arms.

restricted flexibility in the musculature, culminating eventually in an acute attack of back pain.

To do its job, the body needs well-toned muscles and physical balance within its overall working system. Should one muscle group be unable to perform due to restricted flexibility, other muscle groups try to compensate, thus imbalancing the natural flow of motion and adversely affecting the spine.

Being overweight is another problem. Flaccid, distended abdominal muscles place up to 50 percent more stress on the spine no matter how much compensation is accomplished by the rest of the body's musculature. Weakened muscles in the upper torso, neck and shoulders can add another 30 percent more stress to the spine.

When the body is out of shape, restricted flexibility and poor muscle tone change the normal pattern of response. Instead of the natural flow of muscular contraction and release, a stressed muscle group constricts and can remain constricted for some period of time. This decreased flexibility affects all related muscle groups, including those directly associated with the spine's stability. In such a state, the simplest wrong movement at the wrong angle at the wrong time can be the final straw. Stressed beyond its limit, the spine's usual protective processes are violated and we find ourselves staring into the white light of blinding pain.

When examination reveals specific anatomical findings for that pain, a few of the most common manifestations are strain, sprain, spasm or, on occasion, a herniated disc. I want to distinguish between each of these conditions, since few back sufferers clearly understand the differences they represent.

Strains and Sprains

The distinction between strain and sprain is difficult to diagnose, but strain is caused by restricted flexibility in a given muscle or muscle group. Stressed beyond their capability to adapt, such muscles may knot up instead of relax.

When a muscle (and/or ligament) is stressed to the point of tearing, you have a sprain. Back sprain is frequently caused by athletic injuries or accidents at home or on the job, but you can sprain your back just by bending, twisting or lifting incorrectly. You can even do it by sneezing or coughing if muscles happen to be constricted at the time.

Spasm

Spasm, pathologically speaking, is an involuntary, convulsive contraction of muscle fibers. This convulsion may come in alternating waves of contraction and release (clonic spasm), or it may be persistent and steady (tonic spasm).

Disc Problems

Far more dramatic than the above-mentioned conditions is what can happen within the spinal column itself when a specific stressor directly affects the spine. The discs, which serve as cushions between the vertebrae, are subject to rupture. This means that a disc's spongy center has herniated (ruptured) and is pressing directly against a nerve sheath exiting the spinal cord.

Discs in the lumbar area are most often involved when this condition takes place. This is natural, since the lower back bears the brunt of the body's weight and focuses its pressure when standing, sitting or moving around. Also, because the lumbar portion of the spinal system houses nerve exits for leg motions, most often the sciatic nerve is involved. A common symptom of herniated discs is intense sciatic pain shooting down the thigh and leg. There is nothing like this kind of pain. Pinched nerves are excruciating.

While at most only 10 percent of back problems are clearly related to "slipped discs," as they're called in common parlance, most people assume this is their problem when they're caught in the clutches of back-related pain. Like Janet (in Chapter 1), they've been brought up to believe surgery is the only way to find relief from agony. The reason for this assumption is easy to understand.

"Slipped discs" were once diagnosed as the major cause of all lower back problems. Since 1930, when this condition was first identified—and until the last decade—the scalpel was employed as the procedure of choice. The figures are staggering for such surgeries, and so is the suffering that results from many unnecessary operations. Fortunately, the new trend toward conservative therapy, aggressively applied, offers a more viable alternative.

And yet people suffering intense back pain often plead for operations, certain that medication, hospitalization and surgery are the answers. But back problems are usually not diseases, they're *conditions*. This is an important consideration to understand and remember.

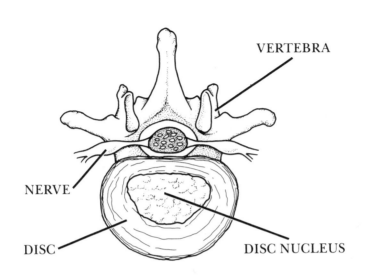

A normal vertebra, nerve and disc.

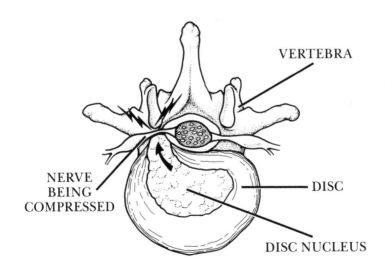

A ruptured disc: When a disc ruptures, the nucleus presses against the nerve.

From a medical point of view, a disease has a clear beginning, middle and end. The clinical cause for that disease is *known;* therefore treatment can be readily prescribed. The general time-frame of the affliction and its progressive stages can be charted. *Conditions,* however, often have no specific, identifiable clinical cause. For that reason, treatment can only be generalized and the time of recovery may extend into months or years without cessation of painful symptoms. For those who suffer such conditions, pain becomes the only real problem.

To deal with pain successfully, we need to understand both its physical process and its mental effects. Both are equally significant in any chronic, lingering condition, and knowledge can change a person's attitudes about both treatment and recovery.

The Anatomy of Physical Pain

First of all, pain is a useful sensation. It identifies an area where something is going wrong and sends a signal that help is needed. From that point of view, pain can be positive. The earlier the warning, the sooner steps can be taken to correct the problem.

Let's say you've been driving for hours. During those hours you've changed your physical position many times without even thinking about it, because when a muscle group begins to constrict, discomfort—a minor form of pain sensation—is telegraphed via the affected nerves into the spinal cord, where the appropriate relay center makes a "decision" based on repeatedly programmed response. An impulse is returned from the relay center and you unconsciously adjust your position.

If the discomfort signal keeps repeating over a period of time, the spinal relay center gets your conscious attention by sending the "message" on up to the brain. Now you know it's probably time to pull over, get out of the car and walk around for a bit.

During an acute attack of pain, however, one in which nerve or soft tissue damage is taking place, the intensity of the pain is such that it relays directly up the spinal cord into those areas of the brain which respond instinctively on a physical survival basis.

Fortunately, the brain is structured so that when this happens, we need never lose conscious control. A portion of the brain's frontal lobes has the power to inhibit all other input from the body. Neurology assigns the function of conscious, associational thinking to this area. Feeling and emotion are processed in "lower" parts of the brain. That's why this furthest extension of the nervous system can control how all other nerve processes are perceived—even their function—including the priority we consciously assign to physical pain.

To sum it up, we have the power to *choose* our response to any sense, stimuli, feeling or emotion. Our nervous system is structured to make that possible, if we elect to exercise the option. Even confronted by intense physical pain, we can handle it rationally and put it in perspective. By understanding that pain can be a warning signal, we can recognize what it's telling us and take constructive action to help the body recover from the trauma which produced that pain.

Ignorance of the body and its functions puts us at the mercy of our feelings. Even those who know enough to tone their muscles with regular exercise are at a disadvantage if they haven't learned to tone their mind with information about how that mind actually operates.

The fail-safe structure of our nervous system won't operate unless we *choose* to activate it. That's literally true. That area of our brain is activated only when we consciously choose to invoke its operation. Until we make that choice, the brain centers its entire focus on how we feel based on past experience. All we can do is duplicate our past reactions, and if we have never understood the body or what pain is telling us, we're left feeling totally at the mercy of an acute attack. Therefore, during such an attack we're mentally paralyzed by our response to physical pain. We fall prey to another kind of pain, this one born in the brain, not the body. *Fear* of pain becomes as real as pain itself.

Psycho-Physiological Pain

Research has shown that our brain makes no distinction between the real and the imagined. An amazingly intricate computer, the brain accepts without question whatever we believe to be true and activates the body accordingly. Thus, when we feel threatened, the body automatically prepares for fight or flight. The more intense the feeling, the more intense the body's automatic, unconscious physiological—physical—response.

Fear of pain *becomes* pain. It's a self-fulfilling prophecy. The mind fears it, so the body manifests it. This psychological extension of physical pain due to emotional reaction is not paranoia. We're genuinely afraid of doing anything that might either prolong it or produce more agony.

Too many back sufferers are told they're exaggerating what they feel. Some, especially long-term chronic cases, are called neurotic. Not so! Whatever the cause, their pain is a terrible reality. The question is: How much does fear of pain magnify the physical pain? Until back sufferers acknowledge that this is a valid question—and answer it—they're trapped in a predictable cycle of pain, fear of more pain, restrictions of activity based on this assumption and the effects of those restrictions. We call this predictable progression a Pain Cycle.

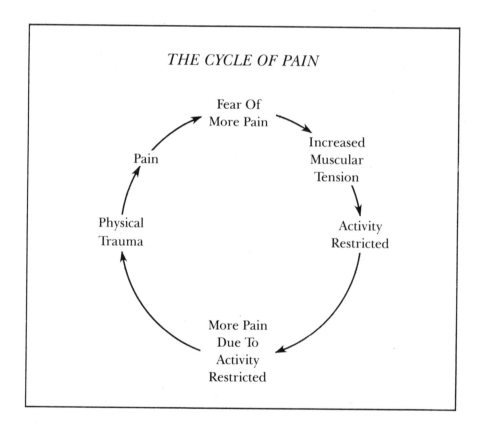

THE CYCLE OF PAIN

Fear Of More Pain

Increased Muscular Tension

Pain

Activity Restricted

Physical Trauma

More Pain Due To Activity Restricted

It all begins with an acute attack of intense, blinding pain. We forget anything *but* pain. Fear of more pain makes us tense and keeps us tense, hindering recovery. Since healing can't happen without relaxation, and we can't relax, we become anxious. Anxiety, in turn, adds to both fear and muscle tension. The result is more mental stress, which multiplies physical stress on the psycho-physiological principle. So the Pain Cycle is a self-fulfilling reality for both brain and body.

If pain persists for any length of time, everything in life becomes focused on our physical state. Just as all we can think about is pain, all we want is relief from it. Nothing else matters. Should this cycle continue unchecked, we unwittingly begin a downward spiral leading to a pattern of physical limitation, culminating in disastrous side effects not only for us but for everyone whose life touches ours. Relationships fall apart. We become isolated, lonely and depressed—all because we're focused on relief from a pain that usually has no clear cause and no clear cure.

As long as we believe the real problem is pain, this cycle will continue. But the real problem isn't pain; it's how we choose to *handle* it.

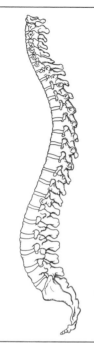

The Cause of Your Condition

CHAPTER 3

Vince was the picture of success. At 30, he was a brilliant attorney with a national reputation, a beautiful wife and family, a house in Malibu and the means to finance an expensive hobby collecting Ming porcelains. Trim and fit, he was also movie-star handsome. Heads turned wherever he went.

And Vince went *everywhere*. He shuttled between Los Angeles and Washington, D.C., like most people drive to work. There was never enough time in the day to accomplish all he wanted to do. Long flights, endless rounds of business meetings and a full schedule of court appearances took its toll in stress, but Vince felt he could handle anything, even the fact that his wife had just discovered he was having an affair.

To demonstrate his athletic prowess, he competed on the tennis court with the same fierce pride that had led to his success in business.

The first time Vince felt discomfort in his lower back was while he was burning the midnight oil in his posh Beverly Hills office. Tired and irritable, he shifted position to relieve the minor pain and continued with the paper work before him. But the nagging discomfort continued.

A warm shower after the long drive home didn't relax him as it usually did, but so what? He didn't have time to worry about it; he had more important things on his mind than a minor physical pain.

After a restless night, Vince was back in the shower, preparing for another busy day. The discomfort seemed to have lessened—perhaps the trying scene with his wife Karen at breakfast concerning his extramarital activities had given him something else to think about.

The drive to court didn't ease either his back or his mind. He found himself shifting uncomfortably behind the wheel of his Mercedes. He was even more uncomfortable sitting in court. Only standing to state his case or to cross-examine witnesses brought a measure of relief.

That evening, after a business dinner, he had more office work to do. By then discomfort had become low-grade pain. It began to get in the way of his thinking. By an act of will, he kept his focus and headed home. When the going got tough, he reminded himself, the tough got going. Besides, he thrived on stress and activity; they brought out the best in him. Competition, even with himself, was what he lived for. No little pain could change that!

Happily, his wife slept late the next morning and he was off and running without another argument. At court, it became clear he'd win his case. Feeling good, except for some lingering pain, Vince headed home with champagne and roses, where he made a successful plea for a reconciliation, vowing to give up "the other woman."

The weekend was a good one; lovemaking seemed to heal his back. His only twinge came while playing doubles at the country club. As a matter of fact, he took the twinge as a sign of weakness and threw himself even more fully into the game. Winning was a matter of pride.

Each weekday found him sitting for ten solid hours at his desk without even a lunch break. When he prepared to leave in the evening, Vince was barely able to rise from his chair. Pain clutched him like a vise, cramping his hips. Still, his schedule didn't permit suffering; he vowed to keep going, no matter what.

And he did.

Sleep was becoming harder and harder to achieve. Almost every night, Vince roamed the house or took strolls on the beach. And as he walked, he worried. Afraid of doing anything that might aggravate his condition, he stopped playing tennis and began using pain as an excuse to refuse social invitations. Finally, Karen pleaded with him to see me. Vince had little use for doctors, but we knew each other on a social level; consulting me would be easier than dealing with a stranger. Denying that his problem was that serious, however, he refused.

To convince Karen that he didn't need medical attention, Vince made love to her more often—the kind of vigorous, dominant sex he associated with a masculine image. As painful as intercourse had become, he wasn't about to let his wife know that sex was hurting him. He'd always been a winner; anything less than the best was beneath him. Still, when he found that a faked orgasm brought a quicker end to pain, he took to feigning climax. That didn't make him feel any better about himself, their relationship or life in general.

It took four more months of suffering before Vince broke down and called my office. In the interim, he'd talked the family doctor into several prescriptions for Valium which he reinforced with marijuana and martinis. While this combination provided some relief, it also made it hard for him to think clearly.

I advised hospitalization to insure that he would give his mind and body the rest they wouldn't get amidst the stress he lived with at home. Vince agreed to follow my advice—but not until he'd completed a current case.

As a possible source of temporary relief, I was fitting him with an orthopedic corset when a surge of pain breached his limit of endurance. He reached the point of no return and fainted. When he regained consciousness, the issue was settled. Vince entered the hospital immediately.

Surgery wasn't indicated, and after two weeks in traction, Vince informed me that his pain was "almost under control" and that he wanted to be discharged. When he left the hospital, he promised to sign up at the outpatient rehabilitation clinic.

For a month, Vince followed a program of supervised training in exercise and relaxation skills. Then, feeling better every day, he announced that it was back to business. Daily visits to the clinic became too time-consuming. Given the choice between taking care of his body or his career, Vince opted for the latter.

As his career challenges increased, so did his stress. Professional and social pressures multiplied, but Vince ploughed onward, pushing himself to the limit as he had before his acute attack. When back pain began to reassert itself, he chose to ignore the situation. Figuring he'd handled it once and could again, grim determination became his modus operandi. Suffering was his punishment for previous infidelities, he thought, and the guilt he felt for putting his career ahead of his family was once again being repaid in pain.

Anger, depression and pain became the norm at home. Marijuana and martinis eased the tension only slightly, but any degree of escape from pain was welcome.

Professionally, Vince kept his head above water by assigning junior firm members to do all the leg work necessary in getting cases into court. He forced himself and he forced them. The atmosphere in the office became as grim as his determination. Tempers flared often; hostility seemed the order of the day. Still, he kept himself sufficiently in control to handle court appearances—or so he thought. One afternoon, during an important labor arbitration hearing, Vince exploded in an abusive outburst and the judge cited him for contempt.

His public loss of self-control humiliated him. He blamed pain for all his problems. It became his obsession. Karen couldn't stand it anymore and threatened divorce unless he agreed to come back to my office.

I couldn't believe the change that seven months had wrought. Vince looked ten years older than his age; his face was lined with suffering. His posture was that of a man twice his age. I immediately sent him back into the hospital, but tests showed that he didn't have a pinched nerve. His only problem was general muscle tension, sustained by the cumulative stress he courted as part of his lifestyle. And yet the physical pain was real. So was the fear of pain that sustained it.

I knew Vince loved his profession. He loved the pace and passion of it, and thrived on the rewards of prestige and power it offered. But now he'd become its victim and faced a choice of appalling consequences. He must change his lifestyle before pain crippled him permanently. And all because he'd so long denied what pain had been telling him—stress was taking a toll on his body.

Vince isn't alone in this dilemma. Not all high-stress lifestyles are as glamorous as his. You don't have to be a high-powered professional to be under pressure. Teachers, machinists, flight attendants, housewives, office or construction workers—every one of us is caught up in the same emotions, reaction patterns and mistakes based on ignorance of how the body functions. Every one of us is a potential victim of long-term stress.

I'm not talking about the specific muscle stress related to a "wrong move in the wrong way at the wrong time." I mean the general state of stress in which we live, year in and year out. I'm talking about the stress of life itself. It is probably the chief factor leading to back pain today.

The Anatomy of Stress

First of all, stress is not necessarily a negative force. Our perception determines whether a given challenge is positive or negative. Either way, the body responds to perceived stress by energizing itself beyond normal expectations. This energizing process enables us to meet the needs of almost any situation, challenge or condition in our lives.

You've probably heard of people performing seemingly superhuman feats of strength to save another's life. There are also everyday examples we've all shared or observed. Meeting a deadline, running for a bus and catching it, dancing the night away yet going to work next morning and cooking dinner for friends that night—all are accomplishments beyond the norm, and all are successful extensions of physical activity made possible by the body's positive response to stress.

This response is physiological; it has its own blueprint. The process begins with our perception that a given situation is a challenge—one about which we feel intensely. This intensity of emotion triggers the release of adrenaline and other stress hormones into the bloodstream. The effect of this stress chemicalization causes withdrawal of blood from the exterior of the body to central circulation in the vital organs and the long muscles that make movement possible. This decline in circulation at the body's exterior has the effect of desensitizing the skin's nerve perceptions, and that in turn allows us to grasp, lift, run, pull or push with less awareness of effort. In this state, we're also less aware of pain. Additionally, this same withdrawal of circulation takes place in the brain itself. Blood and cerebrospinal fluid are withdrawn from the forebrain (conscious associational thinking) to center in those brain areas which have to do with focusing emotion and stimulating motor movement.

The effect is like tunnel vision. Completely focused on one clear objective, any other priority is swept away. Single-focused, we proceed to carry out the action we want to perform regardless of energy, time or obstacle. What's more, as we intensify our efforts, the brain automatically keys in release of more stress hormones, which give us many times more than our ordinary energy. And this is multiplied with every increase of effort.

Given such a terrific automatic energy back-up resource, there is little we can't do in a given situation. Stress chemicalization guarantees that energy reserves are available whenever desire is intensely focused.

Back in prehistoric times, threatened human beings did exactly what animals have always done when faced with challenge. They either engaged in battle or took to their heels. The fight-or-flight syndrome was in full operation. Adrenaline was pumped into the system, blood centered in their long muscles and they engaged in total physical action. More important, after escape or victory, our human predecessors collapsed to sleep until they'd recovered from the intense effort involved in fight or flight. This relaxation was as complete as their involvement in the physical action that prompted the stress-energy release. And during that period of relaxation, whatever stress chemicalization had not been expended in physical activity or eliminated through the skin via perspiration was processed out through natural elimination. They woke up refreshed, recovered and ready for the next challenge or threat to security. They'd worked out the full cycle of stress, from initial stimulation to complete release of the resultant physical tensions.

The problem we face today is that we don't complete the cycle. We don't have a lifestyle that permits fight or flight; nor does it include the energetic, intense physical exercise which would release muscular tension on a daily basis. What's worse, we don't program relaxation into our lives.

This means that the fight-or-flight chemicalization pumped into our bodies under stress remains within the system. It stays there with a resultant toxic effect. As with any other stimulant or depressant, dosage becomes crucial. You can overdose on stress chemicalization the same way you can on any other drug. One martini may relax you, two may make you feel euphoric but, depending on your body's response, three can make you drunk. If not eliminated through physical activity and relaxation, stress chemicalization has similar serious side effects. It becomes a toxin in the body, resulting in muscle tension, decreased perception and decreased ability to think consciously and/or creatively. This is because it keeps the body in a fight/flight status all the time.

Sustained tension constricts the muscles involved in fight or flight, specifically the muscles of the shoulders, arms, back, hips and legs. Continued constriction can easily prove the primary cause of eventual back strain, sprain or spasm.

And what about the effect of sustained stress within the brain itself? Remember, under stress, blood is withdrawn from the conscious associational thinking area—the furthest extension of the nervous system which has the power to inhibit any other nerve messages from the body. With this brain area given low priority as to circulation, our mental focus is strictly on sensation, emotion and past experience. The likelihood of creative thinking is slight; all we can do is repeat past patterns.

In effect, immediate stress eliminates the possibility of creative, alternative-oriented thinking and locks us in on what we already know—the past. The continued presence of stress chemicalization in the body sustains that state of "disconnection" and results in mental confusion, overly emotional reactions, negativity based on ineffective behavior and, quite often, insomnia, lack of energy and a general feeling of melancholia.

In a society that puts a premium on repressing spontaneous expression of feeling, most of us frequently find ourselves in emotional stress with no "acceptable" outlet for the expression of those feelings. This, too, counts as stress. Suppressed anger is still anger; suppressed resentment is still resentment; fear, whether expressed or not, is still fear. All such intense emotions produce stress chemicalization.

Vince's conditioned beliefs made him feel it was wrong to express his pain. That kept him from doing anything to relieve it. He felt it was unmanly not to perform sexually, so he went on until even that, too, became part of his problem. Because he felt he had to be a winner, he almost lost everything. His beliefs, his habits and his basic attitudes made a back condition almost inevitable. His lack of education about body basics and the effects of stress were killing him. But beyond any other consideration, Vince didn't realize that relaxation is as important to physical well-being as exercise. As long as our minds are tense, our bodies will be, too.

In any given day, most of us are stressed repeatedly by some sort of change, challenge or conflict. Whenever we feel intensely about something, a new release of stress hormones is pumped into our bodies. On and on it goes, day after day, year in, year out, building and multiplying until it becomes our very way of life.

The Cycle of Destructive Stress

Ignorance, repressive attitudes toward expression of emotion, lack of physical exercise and lack of relaxation can all result in a cumulative cycle of destructive stress. This cycle is usually triggered by an intense emotional reaction to a threat of danger or a fear of loss.

This is a closed-circle situation, a kind of locked-in negative spiral with increasingly dangerous effects upon the body. The more intense the feeling, the more destructive the effects of stress, especially if that feeling is denied or goes unresolved.

We deny our guilt and grief, our rage and hostility, our fear. We grin and bear it or mask our feelings with apparent indifference, neither of which changes what is happening within our bodies. Stress is stress. No wonder the society we live in has so many problems—it's filled with people who are so

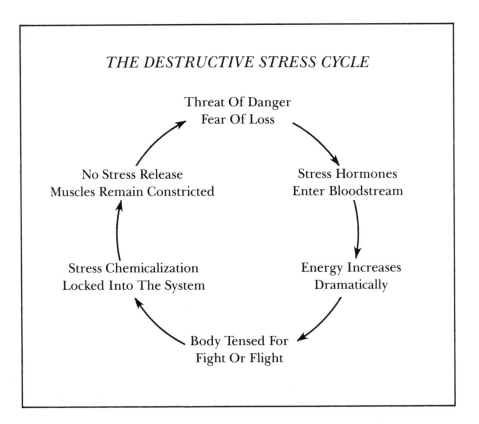

THE DESTRUCTIVE STRESS CYCLE

Threat Of Danger
Fear Of Loss

No Stress Release
Muscles Remain Constricted

Stress Hormones
Enter Bloodstream

Stress Chemicalization
Locked Into The System

Energy Increases
Dramatically

Body Tensed For
Fight Or Flight

overwhelmed with the effects of cumulative, destructive stress that they literally can't think.

Stress affects us physically by constricting muscles, thus limiting our flexibility. Mentally, our inability to think locks us in on our limitations. This is the process of psycho-physiological pain from the destructive stress cycle; they go hand in hand.

Lingering destructive stress is the single common denominator in all chronic back conditions. As the saying goes, "A chain is no stronger than its weakest link." Anatomically and statistically, the back is likely to succumb first.

But destructive stress isn't the only culprit. Bad habits and life's expected wear and tear play their part as well. Let's review them.

Aging

Generally speaking, the older we get, the less we exercise. This is a big mistake because the aging process is intimately connected with muscle tone. As that tone becomes loose, more than muscle is affected. Within the spine, the discs cushioning the vertebrae are also affected by aging. Made up of collagen and mucal polysaccharides, both of which have a high moisture content, discs tend to shrink with age. Their moisture content decreases, and they lose their resiliency. The result: disc problems. As a matter of fact, some researchers contend that early "disc degeneration" actually represents a kind of premature aging process.

Weight Gain

Overweight is another condition that affects the spine. Fat distends the abdomen, weakening its muscles and putting pressure on the back and spine.

Posture

At any age or weight, poor posture also stresses the spine. As time passes, the whole spinal column reshapes itself to accommodate such stress, placing undue tension on the entire spine.

Standing, Walking, Sitting and Sleeping

Any movement, if habitually incorrect, can contribute to back problems. On a cumulative basis, for instance, sloppy posture is magnified in motion. Walking splay-footed with toes turned outward focuses the body's weight on the heels and guarantees muscle imbalance all the way up the legs to the hips and spine. Long periods of time spent seated puts us at risk if our sitting posture is poor. Slouching is as potentially harmful as maintaining an enforced straight-spine position. Simply standing erect focuses the full weight of the torso on the lumbar vertebrae, and if the posture is rigid, the spine is extremely vulnerable. This sets us up for that wrong move in the wrong way at the wrong time.

Even sleeping habits affect the spine, especially sleeping on the stomach. This position forces the head to twist to one side, straining the cervical vertebrae and putting tension on the back. Mattresses that are too soft displace the spine's natural curves and, over a period of time, can contribute to a back condition.

Lifting

Like standing and walking, lifting becomes a habit. Incorrect lifting habits result in many acute attacks by stressing the back unduly. So don't do any heavy lifting without warming up first. Even then, don't lean over from the waist to pick something up. Bend your knees and keep your back as erect as possible. And don't overdo it. Don't try to lift too much too often or too long for someone of your size, strength or condition.

Exercise and Athletics

How you exercise is as important as exercising itself. Not warming the muscles up through gentle stretches can stress the muscles. So, too, can overdoing it. Many back problems are related to over-exertion while engaged in some form of exercise or athletics. Even the emotional stressors involved in winning or losing can put backs at hazard.

Sexual Performance

High-stress personalitites with an intense desire to conquer and control often put a premium on sexual performance. Sex becomes a way to dominate. This usually translates into unnecessary vigor during coitus. Many couples live out a life of emotional pain in which sex becomes just another demonstration of control and/or subservience. This leads to stress in other areas of the relationship, and it all culminates in pain of one kind or another. (See Chapter 10.)

Bad Relationships

Sex isn't the only focus of restrictive attitudes and repressive mental states. Any relationship based on fear is doomed to create destructive stress. Parent and child patterns, marriage patterns, peer patterns often fall into this trap. Multiply the daily stressors of anger, defeat, resentment and anxiety at home by those same stressors on the job and you have some idea of how destructive stress affects the human body. Since almost all negative feelings end up unresolved, it's understandable that the stress generated by intense emotion tends to remain unreleased physically as well.

Degenerative Disease

Illness is the natural outgrowth of physical imbalance and/or emotional stress upon the body. Psychological research clearly relates many disease conditions to emotional states. Attitude may become the primary cause of illness if emotions have been repressed. Specific degenerative disease, however, also can affect your back's well-being. Arthritis, bursitis, tendonitis and other such common afflictions make us limit our range of motion, thus building imbalance into the body. In fact, any problem that limits natural range of motion stresses the spine.

Accidents

Falls, traffic collisions and other accidents that wound or actually traumatize the spine are rare indeed. For these there are usually clear clinical findings and specific diagnoses for treatment. For the vast majority of back sufferers, of course, the initial flare-up is often triggered by nothing more dramatic than sneezing or trying to tie one's shoes—the last straw in a chain of circumstance that usually originates in long-term patterns of stress.

Lack of Programmed Relaxation

Whatever the cause of stress, relaxation breaks the destructive cycle and permits our bodies to release constricted muscles, processing stress chemicalization out through normal channels of elimination. Most people think of relaxation as watching television or going to a film or concert.

The kind of programmed relaxation I'm talking about is quite different. Programmed relaxation refers to an ability to relax at will anywhere, anytime and under any circumstances. Meditation is but one example. This is a skill we must learn if we're ever to break the cycle of destructive stress or gain mastery over pain and fear of pain.

Until we can program relaxation into our lives, the stress of life continues. Overwhelmed, we struggle onward as did Vince, downward through the spiral of destructive stress until our bodies reach a point of no return. For those whose internal organs are the weak link in the chain, heart attacks, kidney failure, thyroid burn-out, diabetes or a host of other ills may be waiting.

But for the clear majority who share with Vince a life of stress, challenge and the intense desire to *control,* the back becomes the focal point. Destructive stress culminates in sudden flare-ups of unbearable agony, an agony that can spell the end of life as we have known it.

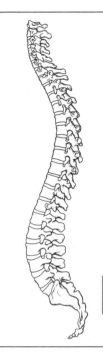

Acute Attack: What to Know and What to Do

An acute attack comes on suddenly, with sharp pain usually centered in the lower back. Of those suffering an acute attack, 70 percent will recover within ten days to three weeks. Within three months, 90 percent of such suffering will have been positively resolved. But none of these figures make an acute attack less agonizing.

Immediate Mental First Aid

Pain is frightening, terrible. But the fear of *more* pain will only intensify it, send you spiralling down into the vortex of destructive stress. So it's vital that you defuse that fear as soon as possible. Remember, your acute attack will diminish. With luck, in a matter of days it will only be a memory. So take charge of yourself, keep your mental dominion. But right now you need help. Get it.

If you're alone when stricken, reach the telephone somehow and call someone who can drive you to a medical facility. Don't wait to do this. Time spent alone and in pain makes fear even harder to handle. If you suffer your acute attack in the company of others, let them help. Whoever comes to your aid, have that person call your doctor. If you can't get an immediate appointment, have someone drive you to an emergency room. If you must call a taxi, do so. Don't be penny-wise and pound-foolish, especially when you're in pain.

Immediate Medical Treatment

Every large hospital has an emergency unit. In addition, there are many small emergency-care centers springing up throughout the country. Get to such a facility right away. Nine out of ten times, a person suffering an acute attack will be examined, treated and advised to contact their personal physician as soon as possible. It's important to ask whoever takes you to the hospital to stay with you and see you safely home.

Use Your Medication

It's more than likely that you will be given prescription pain medication. What you need now is absolute, total rest and quiet. Medication guarantees you'll have it.

Total Bedrest

During an acute attack, about the only thing you'll want, outside of relief from pain, is to lie still. Any physical act, even getting up to go to the bathroom, should be kept to a minimum. For the first day or so, even that may be avoided in favor of a bedpan.

The Best Position in Which to Lie

The best position for a person suffering an acute attack is flat on the back. It helps to put a pillow under your knees. This lifts and flexes them slightly, taking pressure off your sciatic nerve—the nerve that sends lightning streaks of pain down your thigh and leg. This position also fits your spine flat to the mattress and helps relax your back muscles.

Another option is to lie on your side in a fetal position, knees drawn up sightly toward your chest. *Do not lie on your stomach.* This puts more pressure on your spine and twists your cervical vertebrae.

The following are some other therapies that may give temporary relief until you can see your personal physician.

Heat Soothes

Try lying on a heating pad. Heat warms the affected muscle areas, attracting more circulation to them. Warm water also seems to bring relief. We all know how good it feels to step into a hot shower after a tough day or a great workout. It's instant gratification, instant relaxation. So when you feel you can leave your bed for any length of time, have someone help you into a tub or shower. Do *not* attempt to get into a tub unassisted, and if lowering yourself into the water brings too much pain, forget the soak. Take a shower instead. Let a stream of spray massage your back with warmth. If you're lucky enough to have a hot tub or jacuzzi, that's even better, but continue only until discomfort tells you it's time to go back to bed. Respect your "early warning system." Don't wait until pain becomes anguish.

Use Hot or Cold Packs

Depending on the individual, cold can work as well as heat in pain reduction. Generally, heat increases circulation while cold deadens nerve perception; therefore, some people find an icepack more effective than a heating pad. Others have found that alternating hot and cold packs on the affected area brings relief. The only way you'll find out what works best for you is by trial and error.

Nutrition and Bowel Movements

During the first days of an acute attack, you're hardly in the mood to think of eating. Still, nutrition is important to recuperation. Try to drink at least eight glasses of water per day to help eliminate stress chemicalization from your body. Juices, too, are good at this time, but you need roughage as well. Bread that's high in bran content is good; so are salads or steamed fresh vegetables. Stay away from fried foods, fast foods, sugar and salt, since they're harder for the body to digest. The same is true for heavy proteins like beef, pork and cheese. You want foods that are easy to digest, process and eliminate.

A bowel movement can be traumatic in these first days; constipation increases the pain of the exertion. If you don't have a laxative that includes a stool softener, ask your doctor to prescribe one.

Preparing for Your First Full Medical Examination

The more accurately you can define what's happening in your body, the more accurately your physican can assess your condition. Most sufferers don't think about the degree of discomfort they're enduring, but it's a good idea to assign a value to your pain immediately so you can appreciate any reduction of it. On a scale of 1 to 10—10 being worst—the first moments of your acute attack were probably a 10. No matter how excruciating the continued pain, it can't match that of your initial flare-up.

Ask yourself: How much pain am I suffering now compared with the inital flare-up? Keep identifying that degree of pain—when you first awake, then at midday, then before you go to sleep at night. If it seems better at any given time, remember to tell your doctor; this information can be very helpful.

Locate and Describe Your Pain

Pain comes in every shape, size and description. Shooting, stabbing, slicing, burning—all are adjectives often used by patients in my office. A few even indicate that their pain seems to exist outside their bodies, that it hovers around them. In order to accurately locate and describe your pain, answer these two questions in exact detail. Really think about your responses. The more detailed they are, the more you'll be prepared for your doctor's examination.

● Where is the pain located? Narrow the pain down to its specific center as well as indicating its extension throughout the body.

● How does that pain register? Is it constant, intermittent, hot, prickly, fiery, searing, numbing?

Record your answers to these questions on the following diagram.

On the diagrams below please circle the areas of pain and discomfort. Shade areas to indicate any numbness.

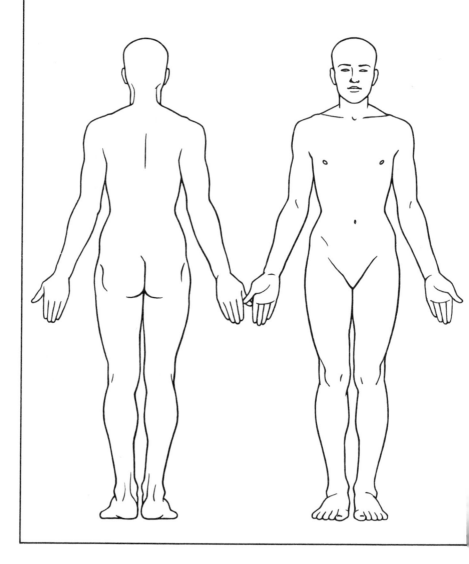

With a pencil, illustrate the location of your pain. Sketch it from its center to its furthest limits. Also write down how the pain feels. Give it a description.

Recording these specific details before your medical examination will make them easier to recall after the trauma of getting out of bed, showering, dressing and being driven to the doctor's office. Since physical stress can numb your mind, this kind of preparation works to speed up the examination.

Your First Full Medical Examination

Your doctor will make this as painless as possible. What physicians want first is a clear readout of your current symptoms. This includes all you know about the immediate cause of your painful episode. If the acute attack was brought about by doing something you consider stupid or embarrassing, don't waste time trying to cover it up. Every clue is important, so if it happened while you were engaged in childish horseplay, overextending yourself in weekend sports or while having sex, tell all. Each physical activity involves different muscles. Knowing which were involved at the time of the attack aids in pinpointing what has gone wrong and what can be done about it.

Remember, don't be surprised if your suffering has no clear anatomical or physical findings. That's not an exception—it's usually the rule. But even though physicians may not know the cause, we can be clear on the effects. What's more, we know better how to deal with those effects now than ever before in medical history.

Still, if you're wondering whether you need surgery—or if you've convinced yourself that an operation is the only way to relieve your acute pain—now is the time for you to think more about it.

Unless your acute attack produces a specific trauma that affects bladder and bowel continence or leaves you truly paralyzed, surgery is *not* indicated. Responsible orthopedic specialists will not even consider an operation until after weeks of clinical observation that would include a battery of tests. Modern medicine no longer rushes into surgery, because it has been found that most clinically diagnosed herniated discs respond to conservative treatment, aggressively applied.

In cases where an operation is necessary, it should be pointed out that surgical intervention has its risks. When you violate the integrity of such an intricate structure as the spine, you could be setting up a chain reaction of side effects that can be as problematic, in the long run, as the initial cause for surgery.

Diskectomies (removal of a herniated disc or discs) and laminectomies (removal of a portion of the vertebrae arching over a disc) have come a long way since they were popularized in the thirties. Today, both operations have a success ratio of 85 percent, and a quarter million of them are performed annually in the United States alone. That's quite a record of success. But what about the 15 percent that fail? The answer is that more than 30,000 Americans will endure surgery this year only to discover that it didn't relieve their pain.

What's more, one-third of all disc operations, whether successful or not, require some form of follow-up surgery. In some instances, a second operation is performed to remove scar tissue resulting from the first operation. During the same procedure, two or more vertebrae are permanently fused together. While this strengthens that portion of the spinal column, it also limits a person's physical range of motion for *life*.

Unsuccessful back operations are miserable experiences and unnecessary surgery is a shame. That's why I urge you to avoid the *first* surgery if at all possible. And always get a second opinion from an independent source. By "independent source" I mean a specialist who has no connection with the doctor who prescribed surgery. This doesn't indicate distrust in the first physician; in fact, it is more than likely that he will encourage you to seek a second opinion.

The only exception to this rule is when a person has sustained a physical wound to the spine from a catastrophic automobile accident, bullet wound or other severe blow. Beyond such anatomical trauma, and the specific clinical conditions of true inability to walk, there is no reason for emergency surgery during an acute attack.

The First Week of an Acute Attack

As I've said earlier, 70 percent of all acute attacks pass within ten days to three weeks. This means that your pain will noticeably subside within the first seven days. If you're still worrying about a possible operation, however, remember that few physicians would subject anyone to spinal surgery until after at least two months of careful observation. So relax your mind and get on with the business of recuperation.

Your doctor is likely to prescribe additional treatment modalities at the time of your examination. You should be aware of what they are and what they do.

Diathermy and Ultrasound

Both of these treatments are usually performed by medical assistants in your doctor's office and both offer some degree of relief from pain. Neither technique causes discomfort. In fact, they're mildly pleasant. Both stimulate tissues under the skin by generating heat, thus calming the nerves and muscles that are causing pain in that area. This is done by focusing sound waves (ultrasound) or a mild electrical charge (diathermy) on the affected area.

Even when effective, the results most often are only temporary. But then, in your current state, any relief is a blessing.

TENS
(Transcutaneous Electrical Nerve Stimulation)

Not unrelated to principles of acupuncture, TENS uses electrodes (connected to an electrical signal generator) to evoke nerve impulses via a periodic pulsing sensation. When this sensation is focused on the area of muscle tension and pain, many patients report significant improvement and extended pain-free periods. Several body sites can be stimulated simultaneously. As with ultrasound and dithermy, however, the effects are only temporary.

Orthopedic Appliances

Depending on your individual condition, there are a variety of braces, corsets and other appliances that give support to your back and may help relieve pain. Something tight around the abdomen and lower spine can offer your back additional support. The relief may be slight, but every little bit counts when you're in pain. Should your doctor prescribe such an appliance, remember that its use is only temporary. Your goal is to be free of any apparatus except your own back muscles.

Massage

In the first days of an acute attack, even the thought of being touched can make you cringe. A bit later, however, massage is useful as an aid to relaxation, especially if the person giving that massage uses a gentle touch. Naturally, a professional massage is best, but a loved one or caring friend might be enlisted. Ask your doctor for some guidelines before you allow a nonprofessional to touch your back.

Those guidelines will be based on stroking rather than kneading your muscles. Kneading can be extremely painful if sprain or strain has taken place. The object is relaxation. Gentle, repeated stroking of back muscles brings circulation to the area, and increased circulation brings relaxing warmth.

Both sides of your spine will need equal attention since muscles are paired in sets. Don't concentrate on the affected area alone, for while musculature of the back is involved, so are hips, legs, shoulders, neck and arms.

Continued Rest

Your doctor will most likely prescribe continued bedrest for a length of time, depending on your progress. Heed that advice. While increasing activity is appropriate to your recuperation, resting before as well as after such activity is the rule to follow. If you violate this rule and overexert yourself, you're likely to prolong recuperation. Don't take unnecesary risks.

Getting Back on Your Feet

Your acute attack will be well on the wane within ten days' time. But you don't need to wait that long to help recovery begin. No matter how bad the initial pain, you very probably *can* walk, bend or sit to some extent. And there are ways to increase your level of activity after the first day or two of bedrest. As a matter of fact, physical pain is likely to decrease with increased activity.

Freed from the restrictions of the psycho-physiological pain imposed by fear, increased physical activity permits back muscles to rebalance their function and reduces pressure on the spine. Given time, continued rest/ relaxation and consciously controlled activity, even the most serious back problem will improve.

Recent strides in medical research on recovery from back problems bear this out. At the University of Miami's Comprehensive Pain Center, Director Hubert L. Rosomoff, M.D., weans his patients off analgesics in days and returns them to the workplace as soon as possible. To many tradition-oriented authorities, Dr. Rosomoff's recovery techniques may seem unorthodox, but his track record speaks for itself. His philosophy is based on a whole new approach to handling acute or prolonged suffering. As Dr. Rosomoff explains, "Our goal is to restore function, not to obliterate pain."

No one has stated the recovery objective as clearly or as realistically. It's on the basis of this philosophy that remarkable progress is now being made in returning back sufferers to their jobs and to active social lives. Using the "restore function, not obliterate pain" approach, sufferers are confronted with the fact that they *can* perfrom the very physical activities they fear will cause more pain.

A waiter who'd suffered an acute attack while carrying a loaded tray, for instance, might be presented with another loaded tray to carry, or a housewife whose problem began while cleaning the house would be told to vacuum a carpet. In almost every instance, the recoverers find that they can perform the very acts associated with the "cause" of their acute attack. If not, they won't be any worse off than they are already.

Other patients might be told to make a twisting, lifting or bending motion that's certain to prompt some pain. When the expected pang occurs, they discover that the world doesn't fall apart. Instead they learn that a hot pack or a towel filled with ice can make the flare-up manageable. Convinced that they can handle more physical activity and stay in control, they find that their attitude changes from simply wanting relief from pain to a desire to get better fast.

My friend and past associate, Vert Mooney, M.D., who is Chief of Orthopedic Surgery at Southwestern Medical School, takes the view that bedrest is not necessarily the best first therapy for suspected "slipped discs." Says Dr. Mooney: "Walking around won't hurt the disc, and it's better for the muscles."

As the most *extreme* example of this whole new approach to back problems and pain management, some surgeons at New York Hospital send patients directly from surgery to the Physical Medicine Department for physical therapy. The majority of these patients are walking and doing water exercises within three days.

The above examples of conservative therapy, aggressively applied, all come from carefully controlled clinical experimentation and treatment. I've presented them to encourage you, not to suggest that you engage in any such unsupervised exertion. But you *can* profit from the knowledge that carefully controlled physical activity and/or exercise can increase your level of activity and speed recovery.

With this in mind, you can begin the following recovery procedures. Remember that as long as you rest before and after such activity, as long as you stay in mental dominion during the activity, you'll be just fine. The sooner you begin, the better. The longer you stay out of life's mainstream, the harder it is to get back into it.

But start slowly. Your body's current condition needs to be respected. You may not be ready to start a program of physical exercise per se, but for openers you can stretch-test your muscles.

Taking the Stretch-Test

At the beginning of recovery, you need to get a feel for exactly which motions are easy, which hurt and which hurt too much. To ascertain this information, you can stretch-test each motion in turn—and you can do it in bed.

A stretch-test is consciously controlled movement, however minor, in which a muscle is slowly contracted, then slowly released. Underscore the word *slowly* in your mind. This is a disciplined activity with a clear beginning, middle and end.

To prepare yourself to stretch-test (as well as to learn a valuable relaxation skill), begin with controlled breathing.

The Importance of Controlled Breathing

Deep, slow, consciously controlled breathing relaxes the entire body. As a matter of fact, when we choose to control our breathing, we're taking charge of the nervous system by activating our brain's conscious associative thinking area, which in turn can inhibit every "lower nerve response," including pain.

This skill is simple. First, exhale all the air from your body, pushing your stomach outward to fully empty your lungs. Now, hold your breath for three seconds, then inhale slowly through your nose, taking in all the air you can. Once your lungs are full, hold your breath—again for three seconds. Then slowly exhale through your mouth until your lungs are empty. When they are, hold your breath for another three seconds. Do this three times.

Controlled breathing serves you in three ways. First, your body is taking in more oxygen. Second, holding your breath sends that oxygen into the brain, which gets priority on any oxygen in the body. Third, the mind is in charge, thus the body's sense-input calms and constricted muscles relax. It is this relaxation factor which is most important right now.

Go by the Rules

You'll be stretch-testing as many basic natural movements as you can—bending knees, extending arms, turning over, sitting up, lying back, etc. Repetition isn't necessary. What's important is to find out if you can do the movements at all. There are four ground rules:

● Before and after each stretch-test, do three controlled breath repetitions.

● Stay in charge of each stretch-test from the second it starts until it's completed. Consciously control it. Think "beginning, middle, end."

● Expect some discomfort along the way. If it only hurts a little, continue. A good rule of thumb that I always tell my pateints is, "Let pain be your guide." If it hurts too much, you're *doing* too much. So if it hurts a lot, stop. But don't stop with a jerk and collapse. Slowly return to your original position and do controlled breathing for muscle release and relaxation.

● On the 1-to-10 scale, evaluate each tested motion. Make a reevaluation each time you stretch-test. Note your progress.

Now for the test. You'll be starting with leg stretches, although you will *not* be doing straight-leg stretches yet. For this movement, flexing (bending) is easier. Gently follow these seven steps:

1. Lie flat on your back in bed, and begin controlled breathing. *Slowly* bend your left knee, bringing your heel back toward your buttocks. Keep your foot flat on the bed. When you've reached your limit of motion, *slowly* return to your original position, flat on the mattress. Do another three repetitions of controlled breathing to recenter yourself, then repeat the exercise, this time with the right leg.

2. Turn your head to the left as far as possible. Return to your original position, then turn your head to the right as far as possible and return to the original position.

3. Raise your head as far as you can. Do not lift your shoulders. Then return to your original position.
4. Lift your shoulders from the bed as far as you can and return to the original position.
5. Raise your entire torso to a half-sitting position and return to the original position.
6. Bring your left arm straight out to the side and up as far beyond shoulder height as possible. Return it to the original position. Do the same with your right arm.
7. Turn onto your left side. Return to lying in a flat position. Then turn onto your right side.

When you can sit on a chair, test your range of motion in all sitting-up positions, turning while seated, bending forward, doing arm movements, etc.

As soon as you can lie on the floor, stretch-test in that position, remembering that just getting down to the floor and back up again is good exercise.

When you can stand for longer periods, stretch-test motions like turning the body, bending, raising your arms, etc. As soon as you can walk comfortably, stretch-test how far you can walk comfortably to and from homebase.

Again, before *each* stretch-test, do three repetitions of controlled breathing. While doing the stretch-test, stay mentally in charge—consciously control the beginning, middle and end of each motion. After each stretch-test, do three more repetitions of controlled breathing to relax.

Use the stretch-testing approach to ascertain range of motion in all normal activities from dressing yourself to cooking dinner. Approached in this way, you'll be consciously controlling each action; therefore, you'll be able to make progress more rapidly and with less pain.

If you haven't had an acute attack, stretch-testing may sound deceptively simple. But for anyone who has suffered an acute attack or who's recovering from one right now, stretch-testing may sound very challenging indeed. The point is that doing this kind of controlled exercise gives sufferers the assurance that physical motion is possible, thus encouraging them to make further efforts toward expanding their level of activity. It's a kind of Revolving Reward System. They discover that the more activity they consciously control, the less pain they feel.

Stretch-test throughout the day, whenever the opportunity arises. Use the in-bed tests before getting up in the morning and again when you settle in for the night. Whenever sitting or standing, stretch-test your range of motion. The more you do, the easier the stretching becomes. Soon you'll be ready for a full regimen of doctor-prescribed exercise to tone the muscles involved to an even higher level of recovery.

Attitudes That Lead Toward Recovery

Wanting to get better *leads* to getting better. Being willing to take responsibility for defusing fear of pain gives you the winning edge. Taking conscious control of a physical activity makes that activity possible with a minimum of discomfort. Keep in mind that in the first week following an acute attack, your goal is not to obliterate pain but to ease your pain and to restore function. Only increased activity alternated with relaxation can diminish physical pain. Keep extending your level of activity and get off medication as soon as possible.

Most of all, understand what your acute attack was telling you: It's time to examine how the cycle of unbroken destructive stress puts your spine in jeopardy. Yes, it will be important to establish and follow a regular program of physical conditioning to keep your back muscles well-toned so you won't have to go through another painful episode. But it's just as important that you start exercising mental mastery over the rest of life's problems that keep your body's muscles constricted. Mental mastery begins with programmed relaxation.

Had Vince understood what his growing pain was telling him, he could have broken his cycle of destructive stress with programmed relaxation. He could have been spared a final acute attack that left him confronting such catastrophic choices.

Janet, from Chapter 1, need not have allowed fear of pain to become more real than pain itself. That fear propelled her into two surgeries and crippling agony.

As with Janet, an acute attack doesn't always resolve itself in ten days, or three weeks or even months. For such chronic sufferers, years of undiminished pain may pass without significant recovery. For them, getting better is far more difficult because of what prolonged pain does to the mind as well as the body. Until they acknowledge how that pain has warped their lives, recovery can remain a very distant dream.

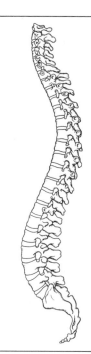

Chronic Conditions— What Happens If the Pain Continues

CHAPTER 5

When the pain of an acute attack has not been alleviated after three months, a sufferer is said to have a chronic condition. Chronic means "lingering and/or recurring," and there is little in life more terrible than being told you suffer such a condition. For one thing, the emotional pain involved in accepting that diagnosis usually rivals the intensity of the physical pain itself. Imagine how it must feel to be told that your pain cannot be explained—and what's more, that it might always be with you.

For such people, pain becomes their entire focus, getting relief from that pain their only object. For some, the pain will fluctuate. For others it will be constant. For a few, it will worsen to the point where they rarely leave their beds. Chronic sufferers find themselves caught in an appalling progression toward isolation—one that includes not only reduced activity but loss of wages, social exclusion, lack of self-esteem and unrelenting fear.

Some can still function in the workplace, but with limitations. As time passes, however, pain can become an obsession and nothing, not even earning a living, can be tolerated if there's a chance it might make that pain worse. It becomes easier to allow medical insurance and disability compensation to provide some degree of security. In Sweden, which has one of the world's most liberal compensation benefit plans, disabilities of the lower back are the single largest cause for collecting pensions on early retirement.

The mental effects of chronic pain—depression and denial—are as disastrous as the physical. Depression results from a continuing hopeless situation. Denial involves two components: first, a refusal to acknowledge that the pain could have any psychological elements, and second, a refusal to believe that there is any problem in life outside of pain. Never mind that you're out of work, that you don't get along with your spouse, that your kids avoid your company and your friends have deserted you. Nothing is wrong except the pain which lingers, regardless of treatment, for months on end.

But before we go any further, I want to assure you that there are many successful recoveries from chronic pain. Thousands master the pain resulting from degenerative disease, injury or unsuccessful surgery and go on to lead full and happy lives. This is partly because the pain that results from such clinically identifiable conditions is easier to understand and accept.

But the vast majority of back-related chronic conditions have *no* specific anatomical causes and no specific prognosis for recovery. With the continuing absence of an identifiable cause, incapacitation and prolonged pain are incredibly hard to deal with.

Why does pain continue with no apparent clinical cause? If there are no specific anatomical malfunctions that we are aware of, the cause for chronic pain may originate on other than a physical level. Confronted with physical suffering, we suffer mentally. This can't be avoided; our nervous system insures that what the body feels will be relayed to the mind, and how the mind reacts will manifest as feeling in the body.

The Pain-Sustained-by-Stress Cycle

The initial incident or accident, of course, really does affect the back. There is tissue damage resulting in pain. Pain causes anxiety and anxiety adds stress, causing muscle constriction. Muscular tension, in turn, blocks healing, and—when we fail to experience remission—anguish over not getting better brings *more* pain, this time psycho-physiological pain.

Day after day, month after month passes in this state of multiplying anguish. Pain keeps us from fulfilling our responsibilities, and failure to do that makes us hate our inability to manage our pain. Medication becomes our only way to cope.

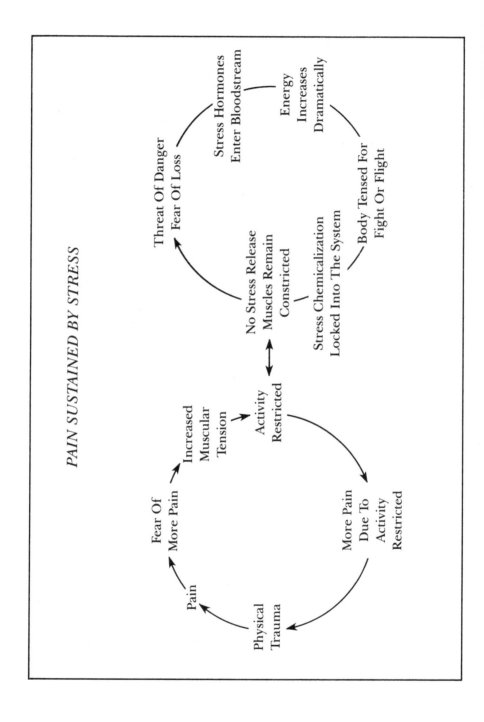

PAIN SUSTAINED BY STRESS

Trapped in the throes of pain sustained by stress, one thing remains a constant: physical suffering. What we feel is real; whatever we perceive as pain *is* pain. No physician would deny that reality. Reinforced by psychophysiological elements, that pain is very likely to get worse, and under this continued strain, attitudes shift. This shift may not be conscious, but it does take place. Our focus goes from getting better to not getting any worse. After months, pain makes us doubt that recovery can ever take place to any acceptable degree, and finally we make do with what little of life remains in our control.

Chronic sufferers are doing—at least consciously—all that pain permits them to do. Unfortunately, that is equivalent to surrender. The battle may continue, but the war is lost. The results of that surrender register and can be clinically documented and diagnosed. It is called "Pain Behavior." There are clear, clinical symptoms for behavior based on chronic pain. The accompanying quiz will help you decide whether Pain Behavior has become a part of your life.

Pain Behavior Characteristics

There are a number of traits associated with Pain Behavior. They are standard patterns of personality change in chronic sufferers. Read them with an open mind; there is truth here whether you choose to admit it or not.

If you're *not* a chronic sufferer, but living or working with someone who is, you'll recognize the changes pain has caused in that person's personality. With sufficient empathy—shared awareness—you may be able to aid your friend, co-worker or loved one in accepting the reality of that person's Pain Behavior.

Here are the established characteristics of Pain Behavior, and a brief discussion of each.

Preoccupation with Pain

Pain is everything—the reason for everything, the justification for everything. Life is centered on the physical symptoms of that pain and on getting relief, however temporary. Things like small changes in physical position to ease pain become big issues. Chronic sufferers have no trouble identifying their current degree of pain; they can describe it in exhaustive detail and know exactly where it's located.

What's Your Pain Quotient?

If you have a back condition and can answer yes to five or more of the following questions, you may be deep into a behavioral pattern that medical science classifies as "Pain Behavior." You may also be ready to toss this book across the room, indignant at the suggestion that you're acting any differently than you did before your chronic condition began. But if that condition has lasted more than a few months, your acknowledgment of the possible changes pain may have made in your behavior could lead to the first steps toward a recovery so long denied.

● Do you depend on family, friends or loved ones to do most of the lifting and/or bending work around the house?

● Does pain impair your ability to give your job the full attention it deserves?

● Do you miss work for days at a time because of pain?

● Do you frequently discuss your back problem with people you live or work with?

● Is medication part of your daily routine?

Reliance on Medication

Medication is part of the daily regimen. Chronic sufferers always have it with them and their medicine chests resemble a pharmacy. They know medication inside and out and can categorize exactly the timing, effects and degree of relief obtained. Since medication is the only sure way to obtain temporary relief, such reliance is understandable, but most chronic sufferers would be hard pressed to make a distinction between reliance and dependence.

Anxiety and Depression

Anxiety leads to and reinforces depression. Anxious doubts about one's ability to handle any situation is doubled during chronic suffering. One must also be concerned about maintaining a viable human support system, and

- Have you consulted more than one health specialist in the last six months?

- Were any of those visits on advice from an attorney?

- Are you now receiving—or do you plan to receive—some form of disability compensation?

- Do you find yourself suffering from frequent bouts of anxiety or depression based on pain?

- Has your back condition made you cut down significantly on social activities?

- Has it limited your former frequency of sexual intercourse?

- Has anyone close to you wondered aloud if you're using pain as an excuse not to do things?

- Lately, have you found it more difficult to hold back feelings of anger or resentment toward those who fail to appreciate how pain has limited your life?

- Do you think you're doing the best you can to manage the pain you feel?

having to rely on others can lower self-esteem. The usual effect is periodic, deep depression.

Doctor Shopping

As pain continues unabated for prolonged periods, second, third and fourth opinions are often sought. Nothing is too extreme to be considered, nothing is too unorthodox. The classic chronic case will probably see a family doctor, an orthopedic specialist, a neurologist or neurosurgeon, a chiropractor, an acupuncturist, a nutritionist, perhaps even some form of psychic healer.

Exclusion from Social Life

With pain as a reason, chronic sufferers gradually curtail most social involvement. Rarely do they leave home; and then only for special occasions, taking along medication, plus whatever orthopedic appliance might help alleviate a sudden flare-up. Because decreased muscle tone from lack of physical exercise makes them more vulnerable to stressors in unfamiliar environments, it's easier to stay home.

Withdrawal from Active Sex Life

For most back sufferers, having sex involves pain. Still, many go on with sexual intercourse in order to maintain a relationship. This shift in attitude from enjoying the act to *permitting* it has deep psychological effects. With pain as the only reward, sex becomes punishment. This leads to the development of masochistic or sado-masochistic feelings. The whole relationship alters once "victim" status has been accepted. The sufferer can't help but begin to see the nonsufferer as an enemy.

Increased Incidence of Hysterical Outbursts

With all the above Pain Behavior, it's easy to see why it becomes more and more difficult for long-term sufferers to maintain an even keel emotionally. The more we feel like victims, the more we long to strike out at our oppressors. Physical limitation, constant pain, lack of the help we feel we must have, and increasingly distant attitudes toward us from those we rely on—all take their toll. Tears prompted by prolonged suppression begin to surface as suffering continues. The agony within comes out more and more often. To others it seems like hysteria; to the back sufferer it may be the only outlet left possible by pain.

Increasing Restrictions Due to Fear of Pain

Last but not least is the restricting influence of *fear* of pain. The limitations this fear imposes restrict every thought, feeling and physical activity. Since anything might produce pain, the safest thing to do is nothing. One by one, the activities that used to provide mental and physical stimulation fall by the wayside. The relationships that used to provide emotional satisfaction become too trying to maintain. Finally, the only alternative is more and more bedrest. At least in bed, the chances of another acute attack are lessened.

With these patterns of response, it's no wonder that chronic sufferers can get locked into a vicious cycle of pain. As months pass, physical pain and fear of pain become inextricably linked. Attitudes undergo revision, and so do expectations. Unfortunately, the last person to become aware of these changes is the chronic sufferer. Such people still think they're doing the best they can—and they are, from their own viewpoint. But that viewpoint has been warped by pain. If they were really doing their best, they'd be getting better—or adjusting better to the pain they have to live with.

The mental attitudes associated with Pain Behavior get in the way of recuperation. And as with Pain Behavior itself, those attitudes have been well-documented.

Pain Behavior Attitudes

Remember, when we feel that pain is our only problem, we stop trying to handle any other problems that come our way. Pain becomes an ally—something that's always there to count on. But other problems, the everyday problems of life, remain to be dealt with, and pain will not solve them. The burden of such unresolved problems, obscured and intensified by pain, becomes so great that most chronic sufferers simply can't bear to think about them. Naturally, such a mindset leads to negative attitudes, attitudes that produce negative expectations, such as these:

Expectation of Failure

Since nothing has worked to decrease the pain, we face the dreary prospect of continued failure in that department as well as in all other areas of life. When we believe we're doomed to failure, we act accordingly. It's another self-fulfilling prophecy. We expect failure, we live failure—so we fail.

Pessimistic Outlook

The expectation of failure goes hand-in-hand with pessimism. More than that, pessimism deepens into fatalism. In such a state of melancholy, we accept our powerlessness to change or improve the conditions of our lives. We are now reaching rock bottom.

Conscious or Unconscious Guilt

Remorse for what we've lost is overwhelming. This remorse produces a sense that we've let ourselves down, abdicated authority over ourselves. Confronted every minute by our failure to master pain and recover our health, we begin to accept pain as punishment for whatever we think we've done wrong. Many people come to believe that chronic pain is some form of divine retribution for past sins and accept this punishment as their due. Pain becomes a form of atonement, a psychic regulator. When a sufferer is possessed by such an attitude, recovery—on a subconscious level—becomes a sin.

Attitudes of remorse, guilt, fatalism and expectation of failure are a burden too great to bear without profound psychological results. Yet chronic sufferers find a way to bear this burden: denial that they have *any other problem* but their pain.

One of the reasons chronic sufferers make this denial is that pain does have its rewards. Incredible as it may seem, there *is* profit in pain.

The Rewards of Pain

Of course, from the sufferer's point of view, to say that prolonged, persistent pain offers any compensation might seem insane. But it does, in spite of the fact that such compensating factors may be nonconstructive. There are two of them: financial compensation and emotional compensation.

Financial Compensation

The facts and figures on financial compensation for chronic back problems are staggering. Disability benefits from state and local governments, medical insurance and lawsuit settlements make it unnecessary for almost anyone who suffers from such disability to return to work. And since most chronic cases have no clear clinical findings as to cause or prognosis for recovery, it's almost impossible to prove whether such claims are legitimate or not.

Many are *not,* but I'm not writing this book about the thousands who fake a chronic condition in order to prolong compensation or disability benefits. I've seen far too many patients exhibit pain symptoms in direct proportion to the degree of financial compensation received. For them, the dollar dictates the duration and intensity of pain. Such people are acting consciously.

My concern is for the true chronic sufferers who may not realize their *unconscious* motives for sustaining pain. Going back to work at a job you hate is downright depressing, and depression adds to pain sustained by stress. Still, most of us don't like to admit that being paid for not working is acting irresponsibly. Such an admission lowers self-esteem; we're much more likely to repress those thoughts and concentrate on the pain that keeps us from thinking about work at all.

I'd like to reinforce this consideration by pointing out that those who receive financial compensation do not do as well in rehabilitation programs as those who don't. In a study of 284 patients at our Postural Therapeutics Clinic, 59 percent of those receiving financial compensation for their suffering eventually returned to work. Of the people who had to pay their own way, the successful return-to-work figure was 90 percent. Clearly, those who are financially compensated for pain have less motivation for recovery. There is a connection. Be that connection physical or psychological, every back sufferer needs to realize the negative impact on self-motivation when being paid for pain.

Emotional Compensation

During the initial flare-up, everyone honors suffering. Many of us receive more attention than we've had in years. The concern and sympathy of loved ones, family and friends is heartwarming, and makes us feel worthy and important. They help us avoid undue exertion by running errands for us, taking the children off our hands, driving us to the doctor, etc. Their help permits us to escape the possibility of aggravating our pain.

And when we first return to work, co-workers willingly assume what they can of our physical burdens. Everyone understands that pain limits our performance and if any lifting or bending has to be done, they do it for us. An occasional day off because of pain or time off for a doctor's appointment cause no problems.

Then, as the months wear on, our pain persists. But everything else seems to change. It happens first at work. The caring, cooperative atmosphere gradually dissolves. Co-workers begin wondering aloud about our inability to recover. Some are openly snide and sarcastic. Management isn't as willing to extend itself when we request extra sick leave.

At home, the kids no longer monitor their noise. Our spouse's patience turns into annoyance. Help given so lovingly at first becomes grudging. No matter how we try to mask our feelings, we begin to feel bitter and resentful. After all, from our point of view, we've done our best, sought new doctors, new treatments, new therapies. But friends stop dropping by, start making excuses for not being available to run errands. What can we think but that they don't care?

The shift from positive rewards for pain has taken place.

Since chronic sufferers don't see themselves as the cause for this negative feedback, someone else must be to blame. The world is letting them down. Doctor-prescribed treatments fail to work. Friends and family fail in their responsibility to understand and assist when help is needed. Even the reality of continued suffering is doubted.

Chronic sufferers who don't get better lose the attention that was once lavished on them. Sympathy is withheld from them, and sympathy reads as acceptance. The feeling that they're not being believed only intensifies their perception of pain, thus causing them to avoid doing anything that might breach the limits they perceive. Escape is the only recourse now—escape from all the problems their pain has created.

Pain as an Excuse

Pain is the perfect excuse for not doing what we don't want to do. Pain equals disability, and disability saves us from ever having to deal with the real, everyday stressors in our lives. Some people find it easier to suffer crippling, chronic agony than to confront the reality of an unhappy marriage, employment they loathe or a life that is unfulfilling.

Pain justifies escape from responsibility and becomes an excuse for nonperformance. We've done that since we were children. Illness kept us home from school when we didn't want to go. Later, it became an excuse for not meeting deadlines. Sickness and/or pain has always been useful for such purposes. The pattern is woven deep into our subconscious.

Pain also gives us a measure of control over other people. It intimidates them and makes them feel guilty if they don't respond to our suffering.

Using Pain to Manipulate and Control

Manipulating people through pain symptoms and manipulating the intensity of pain itself is almost unavoidable in chronic suffering. It's an instinctive survival mechanism. The more intense pain symptoms are, the more attention the sufferer is likely to receive.

In many relationships—especially marriage—chronic sufferers often use pain to get their way. No matter how vehemently they deny it, the fact is that they use pain as a lever with which to pry obstacles out of their path. This may happen only on a subconscious level, but it does happen. The more prolonged the suffering, the more it happens, until at last even the best-intentioned chronic sufferer must admit to using pain to gain control.

I'm not blaming these people. To them, their anguish is real. It's real to me when I treat them. I never discount the intensity of perceived pain.

They're doing all they can to make the best of a terrible situation. The options, limited by fear of pain, seem nil. They clutch at straws in hopes of finding that miracle drug or miracle doctor who can relieve their pain. But what they *should* be looking for is insight—insight that could help them avoid addiction to the very pain from which they want relief.

Pain as an Addiction

Pain Behavior is learned behavior. To varying degrees, we've been learning it all our lives. The pain of life itself produces the same pattern. But when physical pain lingers, Pain Behavior becomes our unconscious modus operandi. The fact is, we're obsessed with pain. Even when we realize its destructive effects, this obsession works like an addiction. It's as real and damaging as addiction to any drug. Even knowing that the final effects may be permanent immobility, we still see no possibility of change.

Who knows why we allow this to happen to ourselves? But we do. Even when we see recovery by others who suffer conditions similar to our own, for some reason buried deep in our individual belief systems, we persist in this pattern of self-destructive behavior. And we're not the only ones affected.

The Effects of Your Pain Behavior on Others

The negative changes chronic sufferers observe in others are simply the mirror of their own Pain Behavior.

Imagine how it feels to invest time, energy and sympathy in your recovery, then have to confront failure. It's painful for another to see someone he or she loves or admires reduced to misery, unable to function socially, unable to work, unable to do anything but complain about physical discomfort. How awful to see you either retreat from making love, or go through the pain of persisting to do so simply to prove that love still exists.

Worse still to see your mind dulled by medication, to see someone who used to be full of energy constantly stressed out, tired and incapable of performing actions as simple as getting dressed without help. How depressing for the person who loves you or lives with you to have this pattern go on and on, unchanging. Even if you mean more to him or her than anyone else on earth, it's hard not to become discouraged with your constant grumbling and grouching. And when you begin to act as if your loved one were a servant or a slave, it's natural to take it personally.

Besides the boredom of not being able to share his or her own interests with you, and the indescribable burden of listening to an endless litany of suffering, or long hours when you lie passed out in drugged oblivion, there's the added load of having to do two people's work instead of one. Your incapacitation has created so much more work for the person you love that he or she is bound to feel resentful. Yet that person can't express personal needs in the face of all your pain.

In time, the people close to you will come to doubt that your pain is real. Not only are there no real anatomic causes, but they don't see you making any real effort toward recovery. Resentment, which they've been suppressing for so long, is bound to flare. Then there will be all the times they sit alone, wondering if the pain you cause them is worth the sacrifice. And it *is* a sacrifice; they've become slaves to your whims, moods and negativity. No matter what love once existed, maintaining it becomes an act of will.

How much longer will they be willing to let you manipulate their life? Or to listen to one more "I can't!"? When is it going to be their turn to be the center of attention? If something doesn't change soon, they're likely to start acting out the same negative behavior you've subjected them to since the chronic phase began.

Pain Behavior breeds Pain Behavior. Self-doubt is infectious. Guilt that we can't help the chronic sufferer recover, guilt that we're failing ourselves in catering to another's failure to recover, becomes overwhelming. Those who find themselves in this situation suffer the same sense of isolation, depression and anxiety that the patient does. The final result is rarely positive unless a positive change takes place on the part of the chronic sufferer.

But no progress will be seen until chronic sufferers take a profoundly honest look at what pain has done to them and to their lives. There is no panacea, no miracle cure for what they've endured. And yet others like them—some who have lived through greater pain and limitation—make giant steps toward increased activity. Such recoverers have a different attitude toward pain. They've asked themselves some questions on that score and found some vital answers.

I'd like to extend that same opportunity to you.

Acknowledge How You Feel about Your Pain

Since most chronic sufferers can identify and describe their sensation of physical pain in detail, locate it exactly and know all of its manifesting symptoms, this questionnaire won't explore such areas. Instead, it's concerned with your emotional reactions to that pain. If you've identified to any degree with what's preceded in this chapter, answer each question with the utmost honesty.

Should you be someone living with or working with a chronic sufferer, put yourself in that person's shoes as you review the questions. Appreciate what each yes answer has cost in terms of experience and deep emotion.

1. How do you feel about the chronic suffering you're enduring? (Consider separately each word on the list. You may feel that more than one is appropriate):
   a) Frustrated
   b) Antagonistic
   c) Angry
   d) Resentful
   e) Hostile
   f) Frightened
   g) Guilty
   h) Grief-stricken
   i) Hopeless
2. What do you feel your chances are for full recovery?
   a) Excellent
   b) Good
   c) Fair
   d) Poor
   e) None at all
3. What do you feel your chances are for partial recovery?
   a) Excellent
   b) Good
   c) Fair
   d) Poor
   e) None at all
4. Is the pain so severe that you can't follow any course of therapy?
5. Could you live without your medication?
6. Have you stopped caring about how you look to others?
7. Do you find yourself wishing others could endure your pain so they would appreciate your suffering?
8. Does fear of pain keep you from doing things you want do do?

9. Do you feel totally alone in the world—as though no one really understands?

10. Have you reached the point where you'd do *anything* for relief?

Whatever your answers to the first nine questions, I hope you feel how much *emotion* is attached to your physical pain. That emotion can only serve to intensify your perception of physical pain. This is why I wanted you to respond to the questions. Chronic pain is made worse by the very emotions so many of us deny. Negative feelings are destructive stressors; destructive stress blocks healing.

It's your answer to the tenth question that concerns me most. And here I address myself exclusively to those of you who are now suffering from a chronic condition.

If you've reached the point where you'd do anything to get relief from pain, *why not choose to get better?* Too many chronic sufferers will answer: "But I can't. I've tried everything, done everything. There's nothing more I can do!" Wrong, tragically wrong. It doesn't matter whether you've been shrouded in pain for years. It doesn't matter if your whole body has adjusted to that pain, crippling and immobilizing you. At the very worst, you can still recover to some extent.

It's a terrible mistake to view pain as the only conflict in your life. You must come to realize that it's perfectly acceptable to find yourself in a troubled relationship, to admit that kids get on your nerves, that the boss is unfair, or that your work is unrewarding. If you would acknowledge the real, ongoing problems other than pain in your life, you might not use pain to avoid further disappointments or to escape from responsibility.

Pain isn't your problem. The problem is how you perceive and respond to life. The pain you feel is real enough. But what if it's only an excuse for not taking responsibility for your own recovery, for weaning yourself away from medication, for acknowledging your Pain Behavior and how that behavior has blighted your life and the lives of people you love?

If your pain has persisted beyond three months, you're at a crucial turning point. Don't close your eyes to it! Try to appreciate the role that avoidance and escape may play in your perception of your pain. Your entire life is affected, not just your back.

What might happen if you should choose to change your attitude toward pain? What if you let yourself proceed on the basis that it *may* have some psychological components?

More than that, what if you accepted pain as a "given"? You might as well. That's exactly what your pain is: a given. And as such, you know that you can suffer the same effects isolated in a sickroom and basically alone—or you can suffer that same pain out in the world, surrounded by friends, doing what you know gives you pleasure and fulfillment.

If you choose life instead of a living death, if you can accept the truth that you have linked your pain to life's stress, then you can begin to get better. There are specifics you can undertake right now to increase your level of activity.

You *can* recover.

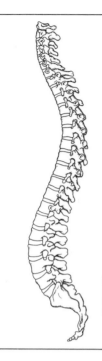

Getting Better Mentally

CHAPTER 6

Before there's any physical improvement in your condition, a mental turnaround must occur. Making that turnaround isn't easy if you've allowed pain and Pain Behavior to change the way you look at life. But the process works—I've seen it work for thousands of chronic sufferers. Still, I warn you in advance: Recovery for chronic sufferers may be a very long journey. In fact, it could even take the rest of your life. But the progress you make will be worth the effort it takes to help you reach your goal.

As you embark on this journey, remember that the only thing you have to fear, as the old saying goes, is fear itself: fear of exertion, fear of pain, fear of failure. That's why, on the road to recovery, the best offense is a direct attack on the attitudes that prompt pain and fear of pain.

Making a Mental Turnaround

Just acknowledging the possibility that you're using pain as an excuse for not making progress toward recovery gives you the power to analyze the real questions involved. Having recognized those questions, we can then find positive alternatives and answers. As the table on page 74 illustrates, translating "I can't do it" into "How I can do it" is the key. The watch-cry of recovery becomes "How I *can*."

Those of you who may be bedridden from long months or even years of crippling pain may have read the preceding and thought, *That's all very well and good, but it's too late for me. Even if I make the mental turnaround, my body is permanently incapacitated.*

That's not necessarily so. Even for those who suffer the greatest incapacitation, progress toward recovery—at least to some degree—is possible. It could be your belief—not your body—that betrays you. Let me give you two examples:

One bedridden sufferer was alone in her home when a fire broke out. Smoke filled the bedroom; her cries for help were unheard. Suddenly this woman, who for years had to be assisted to the bathroom, found herself not only off the bed and out of the bedroom, but outside the house and sitting on the curb as the fire engines arrived.

Another invalid had isolated himself from friends and family so completely that his only companion was a pet Scottie—a dog so advanced in years that she'd grown deaf. One day the chronic sufferer was sitting outside in his wheelchair when he realized his old companion was in danger. The dog was sleeping in the driveway as a truck was turning in. It was obvious that the driver didn't see the dog. The invalid bolted from his chair and raced to save his Scottie's life.

In both cases, fear *for,* versus fear *of,* became the turning point. Both sufferers could no longer lock in on the belief that they were permanently and totally disabled. Finally questioning their previous sense of limitation, they found the motivation to take responsibility for getting better and seeking the professional help that made even more recovery possible.

But why wait for that kind of trauma to make the mental turnaround that leads toward recovery? Even the most confirmed "backaholics" can make the choice to recover. That choice involves looking at your life with total honesty, asking yourself some very pointed questions and translating "what I can't do" into an understanding of "why I don't *want* to." From that understanding can come an alternative attitude reflecting "what I really want to do, to be, to have" and "how I can make progress toward my goals"—at least to some degree.

As long as you think in terms of goals for living life more fully, you're on the right track. With clear goals to achieve, achievement can be clearly measured.

THE "HOW I CAN" APPROACH TO RECOVERY

EXCUSES BASED ON PAIN	THE REAL QUESTION TO ASK YOURSELF	AN ALTERNATIVE ATTITUDE
I can't get out of bed.	Why don't I want to get out of bed?	How long can I stay out of bed?
My back cuts me out of social activities.	Why don't I want to socialize?	How can I begin to socialize more often?
My back keeps me from performing many job-related tasks.	Why don't I want to perform these tasks?	How can I adjust in order to perform these tasks?
My back has limited my sex life.	Why do I want to limit my sex life?	How can I improve my sex life?
I need medication to keep going.	Why do I want to depend on medication?	How can I eliminate the medication?
Back pain won't let me work.	Why don't I want to work?	How can I earn an income?
My back requires regular professional help.	Why do I need regular professional help?	How can I rely on myself?
Pain is too severe to follow a course of physical therapy.	Why don't I want to get better?	How can I manage some form of therapy?
My back pain necessitates financial compensation for missed work days.	Why do I deserve to receive payment for back pain?	How can I prevent going on disability?
I've been forced to seek legal advice.	Why do I really want legal advice?	How can I avoid going to a lawyer?

The Characteristics of Well Behavior

Pain Behavior has clear characteristics, attitudes and problems for anyone in a recovery situation. It takes time and mental mastery to pull away from the habits of perception and reaction associated with Pain Behavior. What you need is an alternative model of behavior against which to compare a successful withdrawal from Pain Behavior. I call it Well Behavior, and here are its characteristics:

Preoccupation with Progress

With Well Behavior, progress is everything. Life is centered on mental mastery over physical pain and understanding what psycho-physiological pain does to reinforce that pain. Every decrease in pain or increase in physical ability, no matter how slight, should be noted as a "win." With pain accepted as a given, you can demand more of yourself physically. Just remember: If it only hurts a little, keep going. If it hurts a lot, stop! It may be two steps forward and one step back for a while, but you'll continue to gain ground.

Reliance on Programmed Relaxation

With Well Behavior, medication is taken only in an emergency situation. Instead of medication, try controlled breathing and other forms of programmed relaxation to manage pain. (You'll learn all about this in Chapter 7.)

Assurance and Enthusiasm

Anxiety and depression are defused by an assurance that comes from "wins" on increasing activity levels and conscious management of pain. Each new sign of progress builds assurance; each new goal attained brings with it a conscious surge of enthusiasm. This applies to relationship improvements as well as physical improvements. Remember, even the smallest win is a gain and should be viewed as progress toward self-reliance.

Self-Reliance

You are the only authority on getting better. Doctors can prescribe and suggest, but you're the one who has to assume full responsibility for your progress toward recovery through mental mastery, honest self-evaluation, goal setting and the physical activities required to achieve those goals. If you seek additional professional help, it should be to find out how to speed your physical recovery even more through exercise, education and skills to program relaxation into your life.

Increased Social Activity

With progress all-important and the awareness that any increase in activity is the same as exercise, you put social activities back into your life. You go out to a movie, go walking with a friend, attend a study group, invite people in, cook and serve a meal. Do anything you can to reinvolve yourself socially.

Increasingly Good Communication

Knowing the importance of maintaining relaxation, it becomes more effective to communicate than to withhold feelings until they burst out in anger or hysteria. By consciously acknowledging your own emotional responses, you maintain mastery over them. One by one, you're restoring and improving relationships lost through Pain Behavior. Feelings are shared as soon as you're aware of problems building up so that those problems can be addressed and handled. This lets you reach agreement with others and set mutual goals for maintaining those agreements.

Physical Progress Through Controlled Activity

By consciously controlling physical activity and alternating it with programmed relaxation, progress is made in pain management as well. A major goal is to return to work or to seek training for work you truly want to do. This breeds new, more profitable attitudes—attitudes that prompt positive emotions.

Expectations of Success

As I've said, every win, however slight, builds self-confidence and self-esteem. The fact that you're making progress and are focused on improvement becomes a self-fulfilling prophecy.

An Optimistic Outlook

Progress gives you the feeling that still more is possible. And optimism based on self-knowledge and self-mastery is never blind. More calm than excited, it supports you through moments of failure. Tomorrow will be better because of the progress you make today.

Looking Better

Typical long-term chronic sufferers look the picture of their pain. Whether they've gained or lost weight, inactivity has sapped their body tone. With the attitude that they can't do anything to improve their physical condition, they often stop caring about their physical appearance, which must be as depressing to them as it is to those they live with. Utilizing Well Behavior, you see with success-oriented eyes and, since most sufferers can still employ a washcloth or a comb unassisted, there's an almost immediate improvement in personal appearance. This in itself is a win of major significance, a symbol of the new direction that's being taken.

Turning Pain Behavior into Well Behavior

Trying won't get you there; neither will wishing. You have to go "cold turkey" in mental recovery. That means making a commitment to choose Well Behavior and act out Well Behavior to the best of your ability all the time. To reach the point of such a life-affirming commitment, you'll need to review the life you're living now. Having done that, you'll need to mentally create a picture of the life you want to have.

I teach my patients to do this through a process I call "Sand Dune Therapy." Here's how you can make it work for you.

Sand Dune Therapy

Somewhere near you (or within you) is a quiet place, a beautiful place where you feel comfortable, serene, at peace with nature. For me, it's a sand dune, surrounded by the silent desert. When I have problems, I take them to my sand dune. There, in silence, I'm at one with the healing, the eternity of nature. In such surroundings, I can gain a clear perspective on what I wanted, what went wrong and how I can make things right again.

Only you know your own favorite place, the place in which you feel most peaceful, most attuned to nature. It may be lying on a beach, looking at the waves. It might be in the mountains, watching sunlight on a rippling stream. It may be sitting in a field, watching the wheat bend in waves before an even breeze. If you can't actually be there physically, you can always be there in your mind.

In silence, lying comfortably, you can close your eyes and see your "sand dune." Surround yourself mentally with each detail. Feel the sun on your skin, the changing temperature as the wind blows over you. Hear the sounds of nature. See the color of the sky. Study the clouds. Watch the play of light and shadow. Feel again the calm relaxation you felt when you were "really" there. Let it flow through you, turning past memory into present reality.

Then, in that calming stillness, ask yourself about your life. Excluding pain, what are the stressors that most affect you now? What do you want from the job/career/profession that you have—or had? If one of your goals is a change in vocation, what do you need to make that job/career/profession a reality? What aspect of that vocation—be it background, education or hands-on practice—could you tackle right now?

What do you want in the love relationship you have—or had? What went wrong that changed things? Was it your Pain Behavior that built barriers between you? What do you want in that relationship now—and can you make it possible?

If your goal is to improve a loving relationship, how can you express the love you feel? Would it strengthen the relationship if you started taking more care with your appearance? Show—and state—your appreciation for any sacrifices made on your behalf. Even if you're basically bedridden, you can manifest your mental turnaround by talking and looking in accordance with Well Behavior. The options and alternatives for your own improvement are already within your consciousness. Relax and let those answers come.

Take each area of your life that bothers you and examine it. Whether the stressors are personal or professional, the pattern is the same.

- What did I really want in the first place?

- What went wrong?

- What do I want to happen now?

- How can I make the situation better right now?

What about your past friendships? How can you bring those people back into your life or find new friendships to support your getting better? If one of the stressors is financial, what can you do to prepare for getting back to work? If lack of sexual expression haunts you, how can you demonstrate that you not only *want* to make love but that you're getting better so you can make love?

And what about your relatives—brothers, sisters, parents, children? If any relationship has soured during your bout with chronic pain, you can improve it—if you're willing to. Each and every improvement in terms of responsible behavior will release more energy and positive expectation into your life.

Even if the other people involved don't respond, your reward is in the fact that you're doing it for your own benefit, not to change them. Your getting better will eventually affect them, and that effect will be positive as long as you consistently manifest Well Behavior. The fact that your recovery has positive effects on others is a secondary reward. The *primary* reward is your own increased ability to enjoy the experience of living.

Setting Improvement Goals

How can you begin a positive preoccupation with progress? Mentally, you might pick one stressful relationship, put your whole focus on its improvement and become intensely aware of your own improved communication and the positive responses you receive. Physically, you can put your focus on stretch-testing to define your current physical limits, making it possible to recognize progress as you stretch-test morning and night. Or you could start taking better care of your appearance, become fascinated with how to make yourself look your best through nutrition, grooming and weight loss or gain. Set specific goals.

Finding out more about programmed relaxation is a good beginning. Beyond what you'll read in the next chapter, there are literally scores of cassette tape programs readily available. In fact, there is a wealth of material you can read, study and do on your own to program relaxation into your life. You need that information to wean yourself away from medication, because being able to program relaxation at will makes the weaning process far easier.

Assurance and enthusiasm come naturally when you're making progress. If you don't have such feelings, act them out. No, that isn't hypocritical. One of the major theories of the acting profession is that when you act out the feeling, the feeling becomes real. This theory works in the same way as any other self-fulfilling prophecy. When we create the mindset that we can handle pain or problems, we're more likely to turn those thoughts into reality. Since both assurance and enthusiasm are mental expectations, there's everything *right* about preprogramming them into consciousness via mental self-talk during moments of relaxation.

Weaning yourself from medication through programmed relaxation, building assurance and enthusiasm—anything you're doing to get better reinforces self-reliance. But there are still goals to be set. Physically, you need to increase your activity level. That means physical exercise is required, to whatever extent is possible right now. Progress on the physical and mental levels will insure self-reliance. Get busy getting better.

It naturally follows that you'll be seeking increased social activity. In this area, setting goals is simple. Telephone the friends you haven't seen in a while and ask them over. Perhaps you could watch a comedy on television together. Or you could play cards or some other game that requires continued concentration. If your current condition permits, you might tell your friends that you're available now to attend dinners and social gatherings and ask to be included. Your options in this area are unlimited.

To achieve fulfillment in sexual expression may take time, but there are specific goals you can set right now to make that a reality. Once again, the first goals have to do with attitude. Building intimacy begins the process, and intimacy takes time to establish. Because I consider this part of Well Behavior such an important issue in recovery, I've described the process of building intimacy in Chapter 10, but for now, making your attitude one of loving acceptance is a good beginning. Your partner needs that loving acceptance and your deep, sincere appreciation for him or her as a person. He or she is bound to have suffered from your Pain Behavior and bound to feel that the "nurse" role has become more important than the "lover" role. Your attitude can make the difference. Start seeing your loved one as your lover again. And start acting that way. Prepare for future fulfillment by acting as if you already had that fulfillment.

Increasing good communication is the key to transforming your image from sufferer to recoverer. Your first consideration is to stop talking about your pain, your symptoms or your medical history. This change alone makes it very clear to others that you're getting better. When you start talking progress and recovery, you'll be seen in a new light. Moreover, once you stop talking pain, you can begin talking about finding solutions for the other problems of your life with the people who may be part of those problems. Your candid acknowledgment of those problems is healing for them, too. The most obvious goal is direct, honest communication on any subject. Since you may never have studied or realized the skills involved in clear communication, it may be time to set a goal of finding out what they are. Many books are available, and there are excellent workshops on communication skills that you can attend as soon as your level of physical activity permits.

Another goal in this area is seeking out people who have recovered (or are recovering) from similar back conditions. Actively involve yourself with them; discover what they've done and how they've done it. If you don't have immediate access to such people, ask your physician to put you in touch with successful recoverers.

Expectations of success and an optimistic outlook are the outcomes of achievement. They are also attitudes you can preprogram with assurance once you've made the mental turnaround. No matter that you may have been bedridden for months, progress is possible—and to a degree that might surprise you. Even if your condition seems absolutely hopeless, I assure you it *isn't*. Just staying out of bed for longer periods is a major victory. Make that extra effort—go outside and sit in the sunshine. With such achievements come the hunger to do still more.

We can do that which we choose to do if the goal is realistic and carefully prepared for by mental preprogramming. The more goals you set and achieve, the more certain you'll be to set further goals and achieve them, too. The getting-better process is a self-fulfilling prophecy in action.

One last consideration about goal setting: *It's absolutely vital that you select your own goals.* All I can do, all anyone can do, is suggest. Each goal must be something you truly want, truly believe in. To achieve that goal takes total determination. Only with intense desire will you find the stick-to-itiveness to follow through. The necessary follow-through means actively doing what needs to be done—not once but time and time again. In fact, making progress in the battle of recovery depends on a regular program of making choices to keep that progress going. Mental mastery is totally dependent on conscious choice and constant, consciously controlled activity.

No matter how physically limiting your current condition may be, your choices can transcend it. However bad the pain, however great the stressor, we can choose to relax. We can choose to be patient. We can choose to trust the body to help heal itself—given time, rest, prescribed exercise and our own continuing choice to make that happen.

The Revolving Reward System

Since even the slightest degree of improvement demands real concentration, control and exertion, that concentrated effort is a reward in itself. So is the attainment of the goal for which you put in all that work. As you track your progress, you recognize success more easily. Success, in turn, intensifies self-motivation. When you do something better—such as staying out of bed longer—that gives you the awareness you can do even better the next time.

If you've allowed yourself to become overweight during your chronic bout, or you were overweight prior to the acute attack, weight loss will bring all kinds of positive rewards. Not only will you look better, you'll feel better—and it'll be easier to exercise. Exercise, in turn, helps you lose weight, and weight loss helps you exercise. The Revolving Reward System is in motion.

Another example has to do with accepting pain as a given. You have accepted pain as something you must live with. This lets you start thinking about living more fully. You take steps in that direction by electing to have friends over. Your effort is rewarded with their rekindled interest. This leads you to think about how you can get out to visit them. Naturally, you do all that's physically and mentally necessary to prepare yourself to handle that exertion. Finally you're ready and you make that visit. The visit is a success and, as with any exertion, you've exercised your body. The Revolving Reward System has paid off again.

With the "How I can" approach applied to reentry into the world of work, you set goals for exercises that increase specific abilities which relate to your job. You practice these until they become manageable, then easy, then natural. In time you'll be back on the job—still improving your overall capability through physical exercise. Strengthening your back lets your back support you as you support yourself financially. When you're economically independent again, self-esteem enlarges your next set of goals to include further advancement on the job.

Doing more and having more is *being* more. The revolving rewards those attitudes provide are affirmative and endless. Once you start caring for yourself, your life will change. Doors that may have been closed for years will reopen. Opportunities will increase and abound. The benefits of getting better are so great you won't even think about abandoning the program— even on bad days or in bad moods.

Any recovering chronic sufferer will tell you that caring for the back is one of life's most demanding—and fulfilling—tasks. It becomes a whole way of life, enriching the mind as well as the body. The reason isn't physical recovery alone; the reason is the recovery of *self*. Recovering pain victims set the ultimate example that life has meaning beyond any disability. In fact, that very disability can in itself become one of the most motivating conditions in life—once it is *accepted*.

What's more, your progress will bring you more positive attention than suffering ever did. Instead of sympathy, you'll get empathy and respect, not to mention admiration. To whatever degree that recovery is possible in your case, you'll be an inspiration rather than a burden. Most of all, those you love will find it easier to assist you when you're helping yourself get better.

Record Your Recovery

One of the best techniques for ending the current painful chapter of your life is to keep a journal of the whole experience. I don't mean that you should author a long essay on your suffering and endless days and nights of pain. I'm suggesting that you start your journal with exactly where you are right now, from the moment you make the mental turnaround. Use the diary approach; date every entry and include anything basic and/or pertinent to progress.

The following is my suggested list of topics. It's very likely that you'll add more, appropriate to your own recovery.

● Write a brief statement of case history, the date of your acute attack, its subsequent diagnosis, operations (if any), what they were and their results.

● List the medical or health professionals from whom you've sought relief from pain, and note the effectiveness of any treatment tried.

● Itemize your medications and list your current dosage and medication schedule.

● Identify your pain by degree (scale of 1 to 10) and locate it as it is right now. Be fully detailed and exact in your description.

● Identify your current physical limitations as specifically as possible. Stretch-test to insure accuracy and note the results for each basic motion of limbs and torso, neck and head.

● Itemize what physical activities you can perform personally, socially and professionally despite your current condition.

● Acknowledge and identify the problem areas of your life (job-related, financial, legal, marital, etc.), other than pain.

- Acknowledge the specific areas of your life in which Pain Behavior toward others may have affected relationships. List the names of the people involved and the current status and quality of those relationships.

- Set specific goals to resolve the problem areas and relationships in your life. Commit yourself in writing to the first things you can do to improve each situation. State exactly what you're going to do with others and within yourself to make getting better happen.

- Set specific goals for programming more relaxation, recreation and creativity into your life.

- Set specific goals for increasing your level of physical activity, based on your current limitation. Be specific about what you want to be able to do and how you can begin to achieve that physical ability.

With case history and previous treatments acknowledged, you'll be able to recognize more clearly the progress you make under your own authority. Having exactly identified your physical pain and its location, you'll more readily recognize improvement when it happens. The same is true for your current level of physical limitation. When you acknowledge the problems in your life outside of pain, you free yourself to find solutions for those stress-provoking, pain-sustaining situations. And when you commit yourself in writing to the goals that will help you get better mentally and physically, you're taking the first steps on the journey of recovery.

However long your journey, however distant your dream, you *will* make progress. Every day, you can measure the effects of increased physical activity and mental dominion. You can evaluate your improvements, however minute they might seem. This recovery journal—for your eyes only— will be a mirror of your battles and your victories.

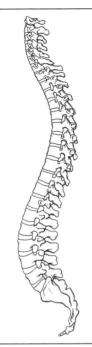

Programming Relaxation

CHAPTER 7

You now know that chronic pain teaches you to behave and react in certain ways. But what you may *not* know is that it will probably take you longer to learn Well Behavior than it did to slip into Pain Behavior. The reason for this is the intensity of the feeling we call pain.

The brain records the memories that result in reactive behavior according to one or both of two factors. The first is extremely intense emotion. Agonizing physical pain falls into this category. The second is repetition; the extremely intense emotions triggered by pain reinforce Pain Behavior patterns over and over again. For the same reason, after we've made the mental turnaround and genuinely desire recovery, it will be necessary to rely on repetition of Well Behavior to achieve our goal of recovery.

You weren't consciously aware that you were acting out Pain Behavior when it first began; it just evolved. But in order to retrain yourself into Well Behavior, you must consciously *choose* it, time and time again. When pain seems overwhelming, your choice to act differently than you did before becomes salvation. Know, understand and accept the responsibility in making that choice. Consciously chosen repetitive action can and will make Well Behavior a reality in your life.

In the beginning, pain is telling you that muscular tension caused by destructive stress has finally breached control. From the moment you elect to get better, however, the pain will be telling you to *relax*.

To appreciate what that word really means, I want to quote its dictionary definition. Relax comes from a Latin root: "Re," meaning again and "laxare," meaning to loosen. Hence, the definition includes: to make lax or loose; to make less tight or firm; to relieve from strain or effort; to unbend. All these aspects of the word apply in the recovery process. Since pain produces muscular tightness and constriction, the key to managing pain is being able to relax at will when pain strikes; to make the mind and muscles loosen, become less tight and strained.

This may sound impossible, but let me assure you it isn't. There are specific mental/physical techniques you can put to immediate use to separate pain from its emotional effects within the body. These relaxation skills work. And they work whether you're deep into prolonged chronic pain, suffering an acute attack, or simply as a measure to forestall future back problems.

Since lifestyles of destructive stress are the primary cause of back problems, programming relaxation is the best way I've found to promote recovery, maintain optimum condition and prevent an acute attack. Without relaxation, pain continues unabated. Without relaxation, muscles remain so tight that the physical exercise necessary to get better is harder to do—not to mention more painful. Without relief from life's stress, you'll never find that sand dune, that place of peace and harmony from the center of which you can examine and acknowledge the goals you desire to achieve.

The Healing Cycle

Relaxation is the mental and physical state that makes the Healing Cycle a reality. When you take charge of your reaction to pain and supplant anxiety and destructive stress with relaxation, the whole negative Pain Cycle is transformed into the positive Healing Cycle.

In this positive transformation, you can see how improved physical function improves mental function. Reduced anxiety and stress permit more muscle relaxation and this, in turn, permits more healing in the form of increased physical exercise. The personal readjustments are focused on getting back into life's mainstream. As the Healing Cycle continues to function, an upward spiral toward recovery gains momentum. In time, the choices necessary at the beginning become second nature. Repetition of

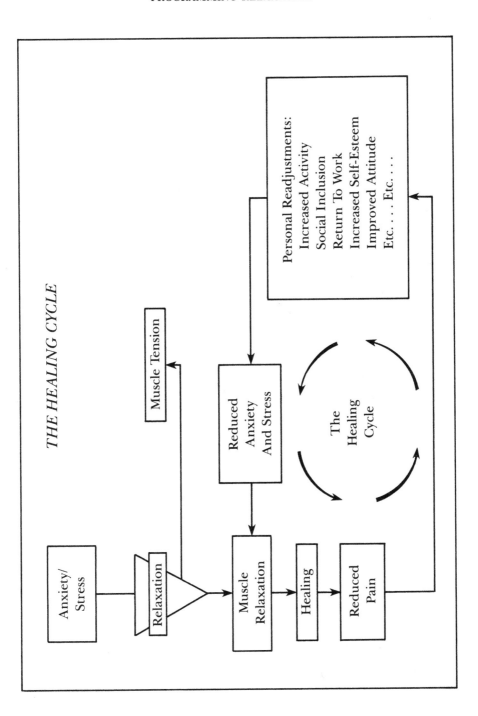

THE HEALING CYCLE

Anxiety/Stress → Relaxation → Muscle Relaxation → Healing → Reduced Pain

Muscle Tension

Reduced Anxiety And Stress

The Healing Cycle

Personal Readjustments:
Increased Activity
Social Inclusion
Return To Work
Increased Self-Esteem
Improved Attitude
Etc. . . . Etc. . . . .

responsible behavior grooves that behavior into the brain's memory banks. Instead of resisting pain, you learn to relieve it through relaxation skills.

Programmed Relaxation Benefits All

Programmed relaxation is a regular, repeated activity which is based on regular, repeated conscious control over previously programmed negative responses to pain. Only via such regular, repeated mental dominion can healing take place.

This will work for you no matter what your current condition. Even if you've been bedridden for months or years, your life will become richer and your level of physical activity will increase. It's true that for some, "getting better" may never translate into full recovery. But being *more* able certainly beats becoming increasingly *disabled.*

Pain Behavior based on destructive stress is the one thing most human beings have in common. On the emotional level, the pain of life has exactly the same effect as physical pain. You don't have to suffer a back problem to be involved with Pain Behavior. Some of you will have identified your own involvement with such behavior. I hope you'll realize that such behavior means you're probably caught up in a cycle of destructive stress that is likely to result in an eventual back flare-up.

There isn't a person reading this book who can't profit from programmed relaxation. There isn't a person alive whose life couldn't be enriched by taking conscious control over the stress of negative emotion and its effect within the body.

The Mechanism of Relaxation

Fortunately, the mechanism by which relaxation takes place is entirely under our voluntary control.

Our forebrains contain a function that science calls "conscious associational thinking." This forebrain area has the power to inhibit any other awareness reaching it through the central nervous system. No matter how we feel when pain strikes, that feeling can be inhibited when the conscious associational area of the brain is activated. Pain, extremes of either cold or heat, extraneous sounds, hunger or thirst can actually be suspended when our mental focus is consciously controlled.

Almost everyone, for instance, has experienced a feeling of queasiness before giving a talk or making a presentation. And who hasn't been in a bad mood before a party he or she really didn't want to attend? And yet, once there, fascinated with what's going on, we forget the butterflies in our stomachs or the fact that we'd really rather be somewhere else. These are examples of how the conscious function of the forebrain has the power to alleviate symptoms or even inhibit them completely for a given length of time.

Another more dramatic example of the same process are the amazing Tibetan monks. Trained in meditation techniques, they have been known to sit naked in the freezing Himalayan snows for hours without suffering any ill effects. Absorbed in contemplation—which is strictly forebrain activity—they remain totally focused on the world within, while the snow around them melts. Their minds control the temperatures of their bodies.

In our society, stressful lifestyles don't focus on self-control. Instead the focus goes toward controlling—or not being controlled by—others. Without the inner harmony that provides relaxation as the result of conscious choice, we're much more at the mercy of circumstances and destructive stress. Only to the degree that we maintain mental control are we buffered from the world in which we live as well as our negative reactions to it.

While there is a whole movement in the Western world toward investigation of Far Eastern medicine and meditative philosophy, it is not yet widespread. Acupuncture offers new vistas in treatment for a variety of ailments (although from my experience it seems ineffective with spinal problems). Transcendental Meditation and other forms of meditative techniques developing out of India have become well known. Gandhi's living example of such calming meditative power is famous. British-American authors Aldous Huxley and Christopher Isherwood have made such thinking accessible to Western readers. Alan Watts performed the same service for the philosophy of Zen. And now the burgeoning human potential movement has synthesized many trends of both Eastern and Western thought into dynamic new approaches.

Here in America, the medical trend is still basically allopathic—meaning that most of our physicians are concerned with correcting symptoms of illness by medication and/or treatment designed to change the body's current reaction to those symptoms. Drugs and surgery can produce remarkable effects. That's why we've developed a society that looks upon physicians as the primary authority for healing. The more we rely on an outer authority to handle our inner problems, however, the less likely we are to do what we can to heal ouselves. Hence, the drug-and-doctor dependence in the Western world.

Where clear clinical causes for illness are apparent, allopathy can work wonders. But the vast majority of back conditions have no clear anatomical cause/effect relationship and respond only in a limited way to traditional allopathic treatment. This left a void for back sufferers until recently, when Western science developed a biofeedback mechanism that callibrated brain waves generated by physical tension. Suddenly we could correlate in exact measurements the mind's effect upon the body. No longer was there any question that mental states could create—and thus control—physical tension.

When we're in what biofeedback researchers term "the alpha state" (meaning deep, meditative calm), our minds become peaceful and relaxed. Our bodies relax in direct ratio to the degree of mental relaxation. The alpha state can be achieved consciously by mental discipline, practice and focused concentration—in other words, by successful repetition. Once we can see the meter indicate the alpha state, we can clearly identify our mental state, know what is going on within our consciousness. Just so, we can also identify what's happening in terms of physical relaxation in the body. Once identified, the alpha state becomes reproducible through practice until we no longer need use a mechanical device and can create that state of mental and physical relaxation *at will*.

The impact of that last statement is enormous when it comes to pain management and increased physical activity. With back sufferers, I've seen remarkable results achieved—not because a machine has been developed for synchronizing mental and physical states, but because a person can learn to reproduce the same effect *outside* the clinical setting. In this sense, biofeedback training becomes perhaps the most effective means we have for programming relaxation.

Biofeedback Training

Since I feel so strongly about the principle involved, I want to share with you how we use biofeedback in the clinical setting of our Postural Therapeutics Clinic. Biofeedback training, as we use it, is a three-phase process. Understanding how this is done clinically will help you in creating your own training program at home—with or without a machine.

Phase One: Awareness

The first step introduces the machine and gives you an opportunity to become familiar with its workings.

What you'll be doing is sensing and quantifying your mental state as well as the degree of tension in any specific muscle group. This knowledge will give you a way to consciously relate a relaxed mental state with actually relaxing muscle tension.

The biofeedback machine measures muscular activity in microvolts. Your subjective evaluation of those muscles' tension will be compared with the actual meter reading. This gives both you and the supervising staff the ability to shape an accurate assessment of your progress in using biofeedback training to focus relaxation in your body.

In order to become aware of specific muscle tension, it's necessary to become mentally relaxed first. This is done through creating images that soothe and calm. The degree of your mental relaxation reads on a meter and is reinforced by an audio tone that lets you know you've achieved mental relaxation. Thus you can both see and hear when you're approximating an alpha state. At this stage, a surface electrode carries brain wave information to the biofeedback machine.

Usually it takes from four to six sessions of approximately an hour each to mentally relax and accurately assess real and subjective muscle tension.

Phase Two: Control

Once you've achieved the ability to recognize your calm, meditative mental state, you're ready to begin the next stage. Now a surface electrode is attached to the area of your body that's most affected by pain. The goal is to enable you to relax muscle tension through consciously directed awareness. Part of this process includes changing the temperature of the affected area—not unlike the example of the Tibetan monks sitting naked in the snow.

A second electrode will be placed on another part of your body, one *not* involved with the afflicted area. This second electrode is to record the body's general temperature. Any change of temperature at either point will register on the biofeedback meter. As a rule, the body's general temperature will not change during the exercise. The temperature of the affected area, however, is very likely to increase as the exercise proceeds. Any such variation in temperature registers in microvolts on the connected meter.

Your goal now is to increase or decrease static muscle tension at will, through conscious mental control. The specific means for achieving that end will be to raise the temperature of the affected area. What happens anatomically when this occurs is increased circulation in that area. Increased circulation raises the temperature even more, thus relaxing the area and aiding in the elimination of stress chemicalization that may be maintaining constriction.

What you're doing mentally is putting your entire focus on the constricted area and using imagery to "send" or center warmth into the muscle group. As you improve your ability to connect forebrain relaxation with focused awareness in your body, the temperature of the area receiving that focus will increase 5 to 10 degrees. In some instances, the increase can reach 15 degrees or more.

The warmth centering on affected muscles releases tension and often brings a measurable decrease of perceived pain. How long this decrease may last depends on the individual. As you practice focused awareness over a period of time, however, you'll find that pain decrease is prolonged. In effect, as long as you maintain a relaxed mental state, your body maintains its relaxation. Relaxed muscles mean less tension; less tension equals less pain.

At Postural Therapeutics, this second phase takes from six to eight sessions, each approximately an hour in length. Some people progress more rapidly than others, but it's vital to demonstrate to patients that they have the power to relax tense muscles by consciously controlling their thought process, and this takes time.

Phase Three: Transfer

The third phase of training transfers responsibility for maintaining relaxation from the biofeedback machine to you. While using the machine, the patient is asked to mentally simulate a stressful situation. Because the mind reacts the same way to either real or imagined experience, this simulated situation puts you into destructive stress, which reads on the machine. By practicing focused muscle relaxation, you then consciously will yourself to release the muscle tension. That release also reads on the machine.

You know what to do when you actually experience a similar situation in real life. Dependence on self is the goal; repetition of positive options is the process. The more you choose relaxation, the more relaxed you'll become. The more you practice focused muscle relaxation, the more support your muscles provide. Repetition of relaxation skills grooves them in until they become second nature and you no longer need the biofeedback machine. The transfer is then complete.

People who really want to get better find biofeedback training one of their most beneficial treatments. Almost 75 percent of our patients have shown improvement in lessening their pain. When you see the meter readings and hear the audio tone signifying the alpha state, it's hard to deny the facts: You are the cause of your own effects. It becomes clearer than ever before that your assumption of inner authority can lead to outer improvement.

Create Your Own Biofeedback

The first step toward creating your own biofeedback is to find a mental image that relaxes your mind. At Postural Therapeutics, we've found that such images are as unique and individual as people themselves. It's like goal setting; until you come up with your own goals, you're not very likely to achieve them. In the same way, until you choose to create images that bring relaxation, you won't relax.

Relaxing the Mind

Basically, you're back to Sand Dune Therapy. You need to recall a place or an experience in which you felt utterly relaxed, then focus your undivided attention on that place or experience, holding that focus until it becomes so real that you're aware of nothing else.

Some people recall their wedding day, others take a mental walk along a favorite beach at sunrise. Whatever you choose, focus on total recall. Connect in all your senses: touch, taste, temperature, sound. Don't picture yourself as a figure in that environment—*be* there, experience it as you did at the time it actually happened.

Or you may be the kind of person who responds best to pure imagination. Many people find that relaxing imagery works best when it's completely self-created. They can create a whole new landscape of their own, even become focused on a single object such as a flame or a prism shattering sunrays into a rainbow of vivid colors.

Experiment with both remembered and self-created imagery to determine what works best for you. You'll know you've found the right one when, while lost in contemplation of your image, you suddenly realize you're no longer aware of your pain.

Once you've found the image that totally absorbs and relaxes you, you're ready to take the next step. That step is to maintain your mental relaxation while at the same time sending warmth to the painful muscle area.

Mentally Relaxing Constricted Muscles

Maintain your mental image and take six slow controlled breaths. Be sure to hold each one for a count of three before inhaling or exhaling. This anchors your mental control and further relaxes your body.

Now you're ready to work your self-created biofeedback mechanism. Your meters are both mental (maintaining conscious relaxation) and physical (reducing painful muscular constriction). Your hands will serve to measure temperature increase. For general body temperature, cover your forehead with one hand. Your other hand will be used to touch the pain-affected area. Your eyes will be closed throughout this process.

1. Identify the painful area with a light touch of the fingertip.
2. Create an image of warmth and center it in the affected area. Your fingertip touch will be drawing circulation to that area at the same time.
3. Maintain your consciousness of warmth and your physical touch until you become aware that the affected area has significantly warmed.
4. Once aware of that warmth, remove both hands from the body, but keep your eyes closed and keep sending warmth to the affected area. Do this for at least five minutes.
5. Check the temperature of your forehead with one hand and place the other on the affected area. Compare the temperature at both points. It is more than likely that the affected area still will be significantly warmer. To double-check, remove your hand from your forehead and check another point such as a forearm or shoulder while still touching the affected area.

Many people are pleasantly surprised by their first efforts at self-created biofeedback. The mental relaxation alone produces positive results. People notice positive changes in temperature from the beginning. They also become aware that pain decreases in direct ratio to the degree that they put their full attention on the process.

When you first embark on self-created biofeedback, expect the process to take from fifteen minutes to one-half hour. But since you will have created your own relaxation image, it's at your beck and call any hour of the day or night, in any circumstance or situation. Repetition is needed to groove in this healing, relaxing power. The more often you do it, the easier it will become. Eventually, it may take only a few seconds to manifest relaxation in your body.

This process also applies to other problem areas, both physical and psychological. It can help wean you away from medication because when you know you have the mental power to manage pain, managing it without drugs becomes a positive challenge. What's more, this pattern of focused awareness permits you to detach from emotions that cause stress. Feelings like antagonism, anger, resentment, hostility and guilt can be defused in the first stage of the process. Physical symptoms such as sudden painful flare-ups respond positively to immediate application of the relaxation/ warming skill.

I've had patients whose positive response to biofeedback training extends far beyond the reason they took it in the first place. Many finally quit smoking. Headaches decreased in frequency and/or intensity. Most noted an increase in their ability to concentrate and found they were more productive at work. And all this from taking charge of how they used their minds. To put it another way, they began living life consciously instead of reacting to life on a subconscious level.

Preprogramming Relaxation

One of the most important aspects of biofeedback training is its use in preprogramming relaxation. By this I mean that you can utilize the same biofeedback process in *advance* of potentially stressful situations, physical activity or personal confrontations.

Let's say you're returning to work after a long sick leave. Just thinking about it can get you all knotted up. You can actually feel your muscles tensing in anticipation. Or maybe you're going to meet with someone who's been negatively affected by your Pain Behavior. You want to acknowledge that fact and bridge the communication gap that resulted. You're risking rejection to some degree, and rejection has deep psychological implications.

For such situations, preprogramming relaxation increases your chances to do what you want to do with greater success and less effort.

Since the brain responds in the same way to real or imagined experience, this applies to real or imagined stress. Because this is true, you have the power to program your responses to future stressors by dealing with them mentally in advance of their actual occurrence. All you need to do is think about them—see them with your mind's eye—and create the response you want to have. In other words, you're *practicing* desired behavior in advance of physically acting out a response. This is done through a variation of the biofeedback process.

If this kind of visualization sounds completely foreign to your way of thinking, let me assure you that it's based on solid principles of neurology, psychology and physiology. It's not a new approach. The popular self-image psychology of Maxwell Maltz, M.D., is based on such preprogrammed positive visualization. So are the important contributions of Milton Erickson, M.D., whose research sparked the development of Neuro-Linguistic Programming.

Preprogrammed visualization is the basis for almost every positive philosophy of our day, ranging from Dale Carnegie and Norman Vincent Peale to religious movements such as Christian Science. In fact, there's not an innovator from Edison to Einstein who didn't first visualize a desired result before finding ways to achieve it. Within modern medicine itself, research is currently being conducted on the power of visualization to focus the body's own healing potential as a way to improve conditions resulting from degenerative disease.

The whole thrust of biofeedback training is to empower us with the ability to turn mental images into positive performance. Preprogrammed visualization has the same result as programming muscle relaxation. Just as we can consciously relax a present stressor in the body, we can learn to consciously relax and therefore better control any future stressors on both physical and emotional levels.

The Preprogramming Process

This process has one ground rule. Before you begin it you must be in the same state of mental relaxation as you were for successful biofeedback. To achieve this, all you need do is focus on the image that brings you mental relaxation. Ideally, you'll be lying down or resting comfortably in an easy chair. Visualization seems to work best with the eyes closed and when you anchor your relaxing mental image by using six slow, controlled breathing repetitions.

Here's the process:

1. In a relaxed state, eyes closed, think about any upcoming stressful situation. Visualize yourself on a television or movie screen, successfully performing in that situation. Visualize the activity step by step; watch yourself doing it all successfully. If you slip up, go back and make corrections. If you imagine something being painful, slow down the image and very carefully do what you know will make that pain minimal. You may even want to see yourself using the biofeedback skill to relax constricting muscles so you can complete the activity with positive results. Visualize the entire experience from beginning to end.

2. Eyes still closed, replay the activity through again, but this time experience it from the inside out. See through your eyes; don't see yourself just as a participant. Involve yourself with every sensation: Be aware of odors, touch, sounds and temperature. As you become aware of each additional sensation, you're etching in successful behavior as well as programming a positive expectation for successful accomplishment. Be particularly aware of consciously relaxing any muscle tension you feel along the way. Take the whole activity through, step by step, from the inside out— beginning, middle and end.

3. If any muscle groups are tense, focus warmth in that area. Relax it by using your own biofeedback skills. When you're finished, do six more repetitions of slow, controlled breathing.

The more you repeat it *in advance* of any exertion or experience that might trigger pain, the better off you'll be. You'll know you're ready to tackle an actual activity when the visualization of that activity feels second nature to you. And the more you preprogram relaxation into that activity in advance, the easier it will be for you to handle any variables that might crop up along the way.

Visualization works because it's a consciously controlled activity. You're relaxed before you begin the process and you end it with more conscious relaxation. As you go through the visualization, you're using the beginning/middle/end technique. That, too, puts things in perspective. You know exactly what to expect of your mind and body. In addition, you know what to do if something goes wrong in the process and physical pain is triggered.

Pain Freedom: A Review

First of all, as always, relax. If pain should strike while you're performing any activity, your primary skill is controlled breathing. Stop everything and take six slow, controlled repetitions, remembering to hold for a count of three before inhaling or exhaling. The control you're exercising will relax both mind and body to an appreciable extent.

If you need more help, apply heat or an icepack to the affected area. Your next alternative is bedrest, but whenever possible, avoid that option. Too many chronic sufferers retreat to their beds at the first sign of discomfort, fearing the pain may worsen if they continue doing the activity that caused it. That's surrender, not therapy.

I'm not saying you should force yourself beyond realistic limitations. I'm saying that you *can* handle the pain and complete the cycle of activity you began. Then take a break and rest. The key is knowing your limits and being willing to extend them slightly every time. Remember, the goal is not to obliterate pain; the goal is to increase your level of activity.

Discomfort, even pain, goes with the territory as you extend your limits, but you must continue. Consider stopping only if it hurts a lot more than you anticipated—and then, don't just stop. Bring that activity to a consciously controlled ending. Never retreat, never surrender. Stay in charge. Anything less is a losing battle in the continuing war to recover.

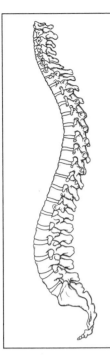

Getting Better Physically

Getting better mentally can happen in a flash of honest awareness, but turning that awareness into improved physical functioning is hard work. Your mental breakthrough will result in a physical breakthrough only when you begin demanding more than your body seems capable of. To achieve the physical goals you set will require improved muscle tone, and the only way to tone your muscles is by physical exercise. Without regular, daily exercise, recovery just won't take place.

But before your condition can begin to improve, you must assess your current Level of Activity.

The Four Levels of Activity: Knowing Where You Stand

There are four specific levels of physical activity, each with its own medical history, general problems and physical limitations. Each is defined by degree of mobility rather than degree of pain.

Level One: Bedridden

Almost all Level One people are veterans of surgery. Some have had a myelogram, maybe even two or three. Most have made the rounds on the doctor shopping circuit and run the gamut of available treatments. By definition, they remain in bed for prolonged periods. Most are incapable of physical activity. Their muscle tone has decreased markedly; it barely supports any movement or exertion. While they might not like to admit it, they've become hypersensitive to their environment.

Feeling totally at the mercy of pain, the majority of Level One people have trouble avoiding Pain Behavior—and are often skilled at using their pain to manipulate those around them. Unfortunately, the one medical treatment they cling to is medication, and prolonged reliance on pain killers often has disastrous side effects. Medication interrupts sleeping habits. Habitual users become lethargic, irritable and withdrawn. Because they seem to have given up on themselves, it's easy for others to give up on them.

There are Level One people who have lost the physical battle, yet won the war in terms of mental control. Such people have heroically accepted pain as a given and maintain active and creative lives while confined to bed. Unfortunately, they are exceptions to the painful rule.

Level One sufferers are people for whom back pain has become not only the sole subject of conversation, but a way of life.

Level Two: Partially Ambulatory

For Level Two people, most physical activities beyond walking or performing basic personal needs are next to impossible. They can usually dress themselves, but need help bathing because getting in and out of a tub can truly be an obstacle course. While most can drive, they're wary of doing so, fearing a possible flare-up while behind the wheel. Some can still work on a limited basis, but this is rare.

Most have been doctor shopping for a long time, and their faith in finding help is fading. They look like "walking wounded" with their canes, wheelchairs, orthopedic appliances and assorted paraphernalia. Although Level Two patients don't require the medication dosage of Level One sufferers, drug reliance can be a very real problem.

They still express interest in their surroundings and make better use of leisure hours, but most of their trips away from home are to see a doctor. They may or may not have had surgery. What they *have* had is an acute attack or a series of acute attacks, and what they fear is a final, totally disabling episode.

Lack of physical exercise and activity have decreased their muscle tone; they feel incapable of much exertion. Continued pain and fear of pain have also moved them into Pain Behavior. The cumulative cycle of destructive stress is at work in their lives, and feelings of desperation are characteristic. Usually their focus has gone from getting better to not getting any worse.

If Level Two people have improved from Level One by using mental and physical turnaround skills, they deserve the highest praise and admiration. If, on the other hand, they've worked their way down from an original acute attack, they face a critical turning point. A focus on not getting worse represents expectation of failure and ultimate surrender. On Level Two, attitude is everything.

Level Three: Ambulatory with Restrictions

Most Level Three patients are approaching the long-term chronic stage. In fact, many are in it. The majority are recovering from an acute attack that has extended over a period of four to six months. They don't share the complex medical histories of the first two levels, but they haven't recovered from an acute attack in the usual time frame. This being the case, they've had complete physicals and medical work-ups.

They are able to walk unaided and generally survive the day without bedrest. Most are capable of dressing and bathing themselves and are up to performing most household tasks—although they probably require help with lifting, or with pushing motions such as vacuuming. Many can still work a full day as long as that work isn't too physically demanding. Even so, back pain may cause them to take periodic sick leave.

For the most part, their social lives are normal and they function fairly well in the family environment. Despite pain, medication isn't needed on a regular basis.

The big issue is how the *fear* of pain is being handled. When Level Three people slip into Level Two, the primary reason is most often fear of pain. Pain Behavior symptoms may already be apparent. Yet it's at Level Three that sufferers can make the clearest choice to recover. The fear they're experiencing may prove motivational rather than self-destructive. The fear of losing mobility, self-esteem and income may be strong enough motivators for getting better instead of worse.

Level Three people must be willing to follow a regimen of diet and exercise. People who don't want to take responsibility for their own recovery put off losing weight or beginning a physical exercise program because they think they can recover without bothering. This is foolhardy and self-destructive. Overweight equals weak abdominal muscles, which in turn equals more stress on the spine. Carrying too much weight makes physical exercise harder, which usually makes these people feel it's "not worth the effort." This is a reverse of the Revolving Reward System and might well tip the scales away from recovery.

Level Four:
Unrestricted Activity, Chronic Low Back Pain

"Chronic" in this instance refers to the fact that back pain is a *recurring* rather than lingering condition.

Level Four people are a diverse group. Some have achieved this level through arduous effort, having climbed the ladder of recovery all the way from Level One. Some have never had a true acute attack; they simply wake up with stiffness and discomfort in their backs that may not disappear for hours. Most, however, suffer from chronic low back pain as the result of an acute initial flare-up.

The majority have sought medical advice at one time or another, yet few have had a complete medical work-up and even fewer have undergone surgery. Medication is not generally an issue. Even so, people on Level Four are plagued with low back pain from time to time and occasionally these painful periods persist.

Folk healers and home remedies are popular with this group. Techniques such as "cracking the back" or "walking on the back" are popular. So are vitamins and special diets. In general, Level Four people have found that relaxation, warm water soaks and/or massage really do help.

Most are able to work, even at physically demanding jobs; they take part in competitive sports. In general, life is theirs to enjoy. In fact, most of the people you know function on this level. They're the ones who can benefit most from a well-organized self-health maintenance program to keep their backs in condition.

Like the rest of us, however, the only time most Level Four people involve themselves in such a program is when there's a back problem to recover from. And that's too bad, because for Level Four people, physical exercise, supported by programmed relaxation, is absolutely vital for maintaining health. Our backs need toned muscles for the best support and flexibility. Without regular exercise, such toning doesn't take place.

Your Recovery Primer

So whether you're at Level One or suffering from the initial phase of an acute attack, here are some general guidelines for your consideration.

They're basically the same for all levels, and they're deceptively simple. Putting them into practice, however, is a major achievement.

- Rely more on yourself and less on doctors.

- Wean yourself from medication.

- Exercise to increase your level of physical activity.

- Get out of bed and stay out of bed for as long as possible.

- Walk as much as you can.

- Program relaxation into your mind, body and life.

- Concentrate on looking better.

- Talk purpose instead of pain, progress instead of medical history.

- Reinvolve yourself in social life.

- Set definite goals for getting better; and work consistently to achieve them.

- Celebrate each step of progress.

In the process of turning principle into practice, everything you do physically counts as physical exercise. Knowing that makes it possible to progress more rapidly. Getting out of bed to sit and visit with a friend is physical exercise. Walking to the kitchen or taking a short stroll around the block strengthens and tones your muscles. In fact, walking is one of the best physical exercises you can perform. Certainly there are more vigorous physical therapies, but intensity of exertion is less important than regularity when it comes to recuperation.

Cooking and serving a meal is an excellent toning exercise for your body. So is taking a shower, dressing yourself, cleaning a room or going to a concert. In the recovery process, being in conscious control during *any* activity makes that activity a physical exercise. All I'm saying is this: Approach all activity, be it an exercise regimen or simply walking to the neighborhood store, in the same way.

Preprogram each activity or exercise. Use visualization while in a relaxed state to see your way clearly through any planned experience. Clearly establish the beginning, middle and end involved in that experience. Know what to expect of your body. Know what to do if you should find yourself in a lot more pain than you anticipated. Use controlled breathing for pain management, and plan some form of relaxation before and after any activity or exercise. Once you've preprogrammed for any specific activity or exercise, launch into it with assurance.

When you consciously control what you do with your body, success is far more likely to result. What's more, when you're in conscious control, the usual cycle of destructive stress caused by unresolved tension is transformed. Instead of being negative, stress becomes a positive force—one you create, control and release at will through programmed relaxation.

The Cycle of Constructive Stress

The stress chemicalization process is designed to work *for* us, not *against* us.

Think how good you feel anticipating something you enjoy—the excitement before a tennis match, dancing the night away with someone you love, the enjoyment of working with people you admire. That's stress, too—but it's positive, constructive stress. And in that state, we work or play with more energy. We're more alert, more single-focused, more attuned to that experience in mind and body.

Our body's reward for a job well done is deep, relaxing sleep. Working or playing to the fullest, we burn up the stress hormones; sleep permits any residue to be eliminated naturally. We wake up feeling alive, refreshed, ready for the next challenge. Most of all, we're aware of increased energy within us. That's because we've released the muscular tension produced by stress through relaxation following exertion.

Constructive stress works in the same way muscles work—by contraction and release. Stress chemicalization constricts the muscles. Using those muscles works the stress chemicalization out of them through a natural process of elimination. The muscles can then relax as we sleep, permitting tissue restoration, repair and recovery.

Sleep itself, however, isn't absolutely necessary to this process. Other forms of conscious relaxation can serve the same purpose. After a consciously controlled set of physical exercises, for instance, six repetitions of controlled breathing will aid the body in its rebalance. So will the mental preparation stage of the self-created biofeedback process. Any form of programmed relaxation helps.

Using stress constructively has another benefit: increased overall energy. When we use the immediate stress hormones through consciously

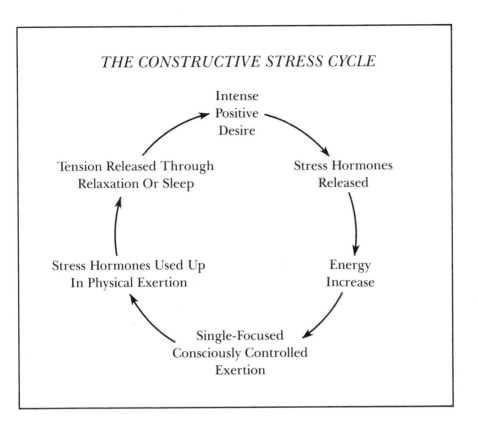

THE CONSTRUCTIVE STRESS CYCLE

Intense Positive Desire

Stress Hormones Released

Energy Increase

Single-Focused Consciously Controlled Exertion

Stress Hormones Used Up In Physical Exertion

Tension Released Through Relaxation Or Sleep

controlled exertion or activity, our muscles begin to release some of the destructive stress chemicalization that's held in our systems. The end result? Those tired, tense feelings related to chronic constriction are gone. True relaxation promotes increased energy—another example of the Revolving Reward System in full swing.

Knowing that all activity is physical exercise, consider this: Done *incorrectly*, even the simplest physical actions can do us harm. A half hour of programmed exercise is wasted if we spend the rest of the day throwing our muscles into tension by sitting or standing incorrectly. An hour walk is a great idea, but if the way we walk puts undue stress on leg muscles, our back muscles pay the price. So before moving on to exercising per se, let's review the ways to perform some basic action habits. Done correctly, they can give your exercise regimen some solid support.

Correct Posture

Spinal curves, within limits, are natural. Extreme curvatures, however, need to be identified and acknowledged.

Here's a simple test to check your posture:

Stand erect with your back flat against a wall, from shoulders to buttocks. Check the space between your midspinal area and the wall. With good posture, there will be some space—enough for you to slide your fingers between your back and the wall. If, however, you can easily move your entire hand through that space, you may have a problem. The larger the space between your midspine and the wall, the more your posture needs attention.

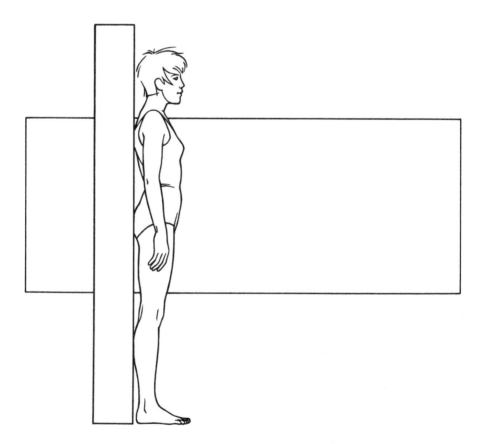

Different people have different shapes, of course, but tilting the pelvis back and sucking the tummy in will help improve a sagging trunk.

To get the feel of what the spinal curve *should* be, try tucking your chin in and tilting your pelvis forward. This flattens the spine more to the wall and corrects the curvature. Now stand away from the wall and keep your stomach in and your tailbone under. Move around until this begins to feel more natural. Throughout the day, keep making that tummy-in/tailbone-under correction.

Good posture relieves stress from the lower lumbar vertabrae. If you have a back condition, correcting your posture as often as possible will reduce the tension you feel in your lower spine.

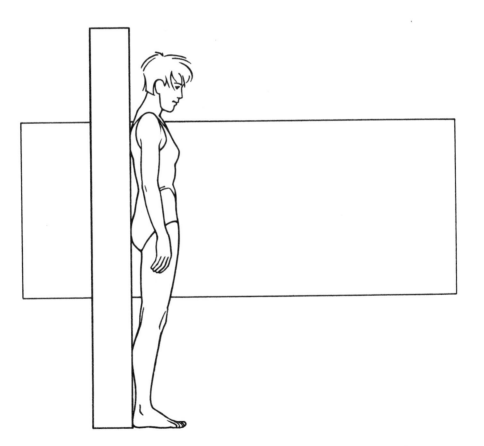

Correct Standing

If you must stand for long periods, keep checking your posture. Your back needs to be straight and your head should be held erect. It's a good idea to use a low footrest—perhaps a hardcover book—for one foot. This shifts the pelvis and takes pressure off the spine. Don't stand with your knees locked, and wear low-heeled shoes.

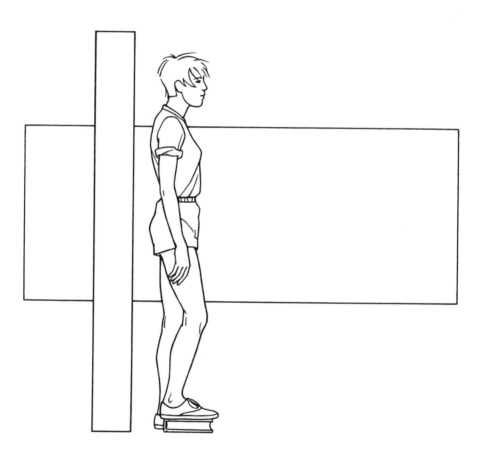

Correct Walking

Wear comfortable shoes. And while walking, consciously maintain proper posture. Stride with the body, letting your arms swing. Relax the body—but stand erect with your head held high.

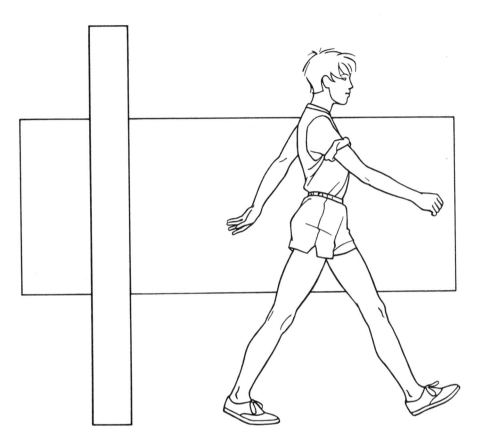

Correct Sitting

Australian physical therapist and author R. A. McKenzie suggests that the most comfortable way to sit is one in which the natural curvature of the spine is maintained. This can be done by placing a small cylindrical pillow between you and your chair back and arching backward so your upper spine touches the chair. This reinforces your natural lumbar curve. In any event, use chairs that support your spine against the seat back, and keep both feet flat on the floor. A low footrest will help keep your back flat. Use chair arms to assist in standing up. Avoid low, deep-cushioned seats.

Should you find yourself having to sit for long periods of time, vary your position at the first sign of low back discomfort. If possible, stand and stretch frequently. Or you can shift position in more modest ways, such as concentrating the body's weight on one buttock, then the other.

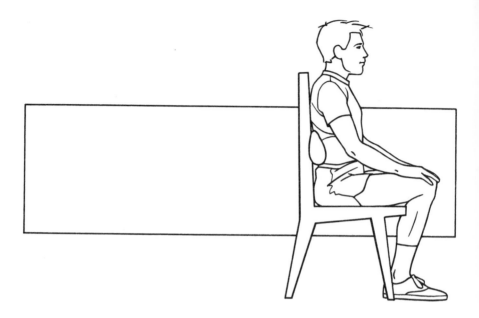

Correct Driving

Move the seat close to the steering wheel so you don't have to stretch to reach the pedals. Use your seat belt to keep your lower spine against the seat back. Some people find using a small cylindrical pillow between them and

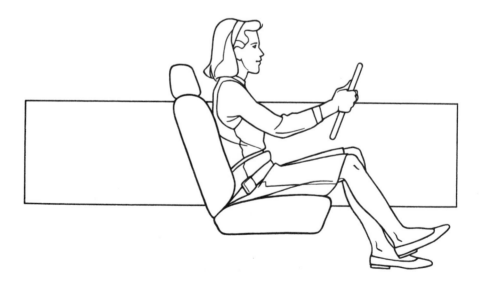

the seat back is beneficial. When you become tired or feel cramped, stop the car, take a break, walk around for a while and stretch.

Specially designed seats, engineered to maintain good posture, are regular equipment in most cars today, and similar body-contoured seats are available in most auto supply stores.

Correct Sleeping

Even when completely recovered from a back episode, you should sleep flat on your back, or on your side with knees bent in a fetal position. Never sleep on your stomach.

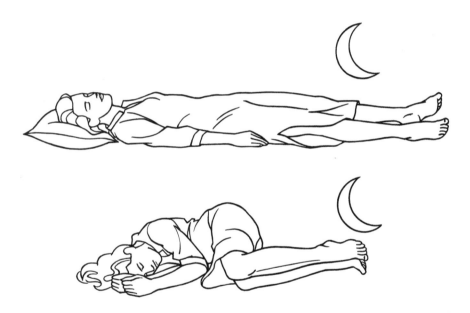

What you sleep on is important, too. Your mattress should be firm, one that truly supports your back. If your current mattress is too soft or sagging, it will allow you to sag, too. You might slip a sheet of masonite or plywood between it and the box springs.

Waterbeds are beneficial to back sufferers in that they allow you to control the firmness factor and at the same time buoy the body while conforming to its shape. In addition, a waterbed provides a sense of weightlessness that's advantageous in attaining physical and mental relaxation.

Correct Weight

The more you weigh, the greater your chances for chronic back trouble. Every extra pound weakens the abdominal muscles and puts added stress on your back.

If you're overweight and currently in an acute or chronic state, I can't emphasize strongly enough your need to lose those extra pounds. Excessive weight puts stress on all areas of the body—back, joints, heart, lungs.

I encourage my patients to look at weight as if they held a scale in each hand. On one side of the scale are the benefits they derive from eating; on the other are the benefits they derive from feeling and looking better. It then becomes a matter of choice between what's most important to them.

If you choose to diet, you don't have to deprive yourself; there's a whole spectrum of realistic diet programs to choose from. The Weight Watchers model is a good one and there are a myriad of other doctor-approved adaptations.

Whichever diet you select, be sure it doesn't give you a feeling of *denial*. Denial is intimately related with Pain Behavior symptoms, so choose a diet that lets you lose pounds while feeling satisfied with the amount and quality of the food you eat.

Correct Breathing

When you're in extreme pain, even breathing can be agony. As a result, most sufferers develop shallow breathing patterns during painful episodes. This tends to become a regular habit pattern even after the acute phase passes. For those in chronic pain, shallow breathing becomes the general rule. It's important to take charge of your oxygen intake, because just as controlled breathing helps manage pain, oxygen acts as a restorative and nutrient for the body's muscle tissue.

Program deep inhalations and exhalations before, during and after any exercise or activity. In fact, every time you think about it, do at least one controlled breathing inhalation and exhalation. Remind yourself regularly to perform relaxed breathing exercises.

Remember, correcting bad habits—even in a small way—is essential for the physical exercise program you must undertake in order to recover. And no matter what your current Level of Activity, you *can* exercise to increase your mobility. Even Level One (Bedridden) people can do most of what I'm going to suggest. There's nothing to be afraid of except fear of pain.

Assessing Your Own Exercise Potential

Let's begin with some specific exercises that will let you know where your body needs the most help. These exercises pinpoint the major muscle groups involved with bad backs, and doing them should give you a readout of the goals you might choose to set for yourself as you approach an actual exercise regimen.

It's possible to do these exercises in bed, but it's best to do them on the floor. Do controlled breathing before and after each of these assessment exercises. (See pages 52–53 for instructions.) Approach each in turn as a consciously controlled activity.

Upper Back Strength

Lie face down. Put a cushion or pillow under your stomach. With your hands palm down on the floor at waist level and your legs still, raise your chest from the floor and hold that position for ten seconds. Then return to the prone position.

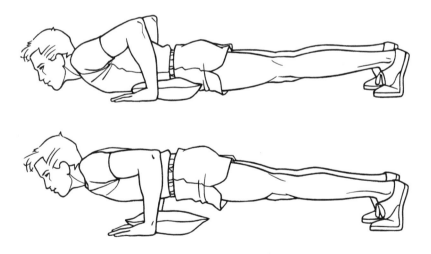

If you can maintain this position for ten seconds, you have normal upper back strength.

Lower Back Strength

Still lying face down with a cushion or pillow under your stomach, keep your torso flat on the floor, lift both your legs and hold them up for ten seconds. Do not bend your knees. Then return to the prone position.

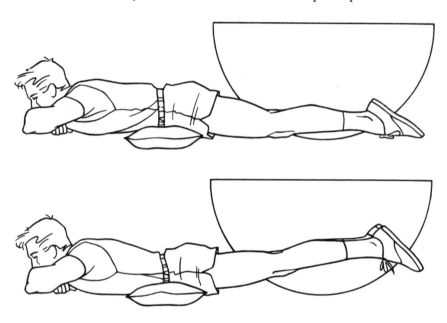

If you're able to keep your legs up from the floor for ten seconds, you have normal lower back strength.

Upper Abdominal Strength

Lie flat on your back this time and discard the cushion. Clasp your hands behind your neck. Keeping your legs flat on the floor, bend from the pelvis, raising your chest and shoulders about a foot off the floor. This is a

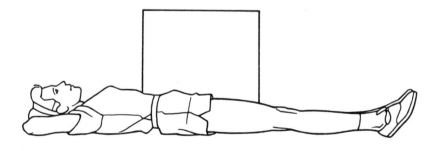

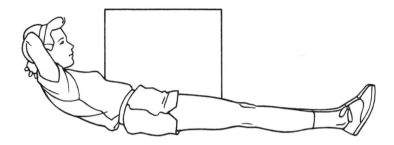

modified sit-up. Hold that position for ten seconds, then return to original position.

If you can hold that position for ten seconds, your upper abdominal strength is normal.

Lower Abdominal Strength

Again, lying on your back, clasp your hands behind your neck. Keep your torso flat on the floor. Lift your legs straight off the floor, keeping your knees together. Hold them about a foot in the air for ten seconds.

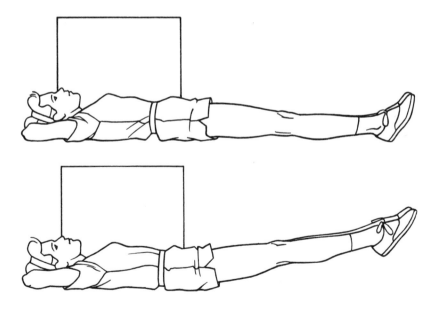

If you can hold that position for ten seconds, you have normal lower abdominal strength.

Your Back's Elasticity

Stand erect in bare feet. Now bend from the waist as far forward as you can—as if you were going to touch your toes—but do not strain to touch them. Hold for ten seconds, then stand erect again.

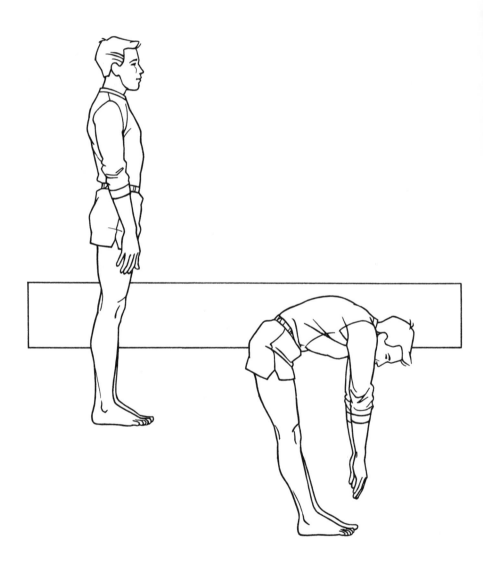

If you feel no discomfort in your lower spine, your back has normal elasticity. If you've been able to maintain positions for five seconds in most of the assessment exercises, you're ready for the kind of exercise regimen I'll outline in Chapter 9.

If these assessment exercises were extremely difficult or impossible to do, however, it may be beneficial for you to spend a few days stretch-testing basic movements of each limb individually, as well as general position-practicing (as outlined on pages 52–55 in Chapter 4). With an intense desire to get better, you'll find your body improves more rapidly than you expect.

Stretch-testing is designed to get your body's attention, to key in the memory that you've done all these things millions of times before in the activities of daily life. Even flaccid muscles respond to conscious commands from the mind. Our body always does its best to support us in attaining that which we desire. So if an acute attack has you bedridden, or if a chronic condition keeps you there, stretch-test in preparation for an exercise regimen that can lead you back toward life's mainstream.

As you do stretch-testing, remember the ground rules to use for all physical exercise and all physical activity:

● Use controlled breathing before and after each exertion, and use it to handle any sudden flare-ups of pain.

● Visualize each step of the activity or exercise in advance so you know what to expect at the beginning, in the middle and at the end. Include programmed relaxation skills in that visualization process at any point where you imagine a problem might arise, so that you stay in charge throughout.

● Having prepared your mind and body for the exertion involved, actually do that exercise or activity from beginning to end, staying in conscious control throughout.

The bottom line is that preprogramming releases physical and mental tension. It lets you know you really are in control of what you *think, feel* and *do.* If you're still anxious about the pain that exercise or activity may produce, it may be valuable to employ several sessions of Sand Dune Therapy in which you remind yourself again that, for the time being, pain is a given. And since you'll have pain whether or not you increase your Level of Activity, why not *choose* to regain more enjoyment out of life by participating in it more fully?

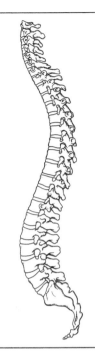

An Exercise Program That Works

CHAPTER 9

The exercises in this chapter are tried and true, safe and simple—and beneficial regardless of a person's current Level of Activity. They're also more than therapy for recovering from a back condition—they're equally useful in preventing back conditions in the first place.

The exercises outlined are starters for a more demanding regimen, one you and your physician can develop as your condition improves. For now, I suggest you do all these warm-ups and toning exercises, beginning with the number of repetitions indicated, and build from there. If some of the exercises are beyond your limit, simply work on the ones you *can* do. The rest will come as your Level of Activity increases.

The same rule applies with regard to the number of repetitions assigned to each exercise. If you find the suggested quota is more than you can handle, *decrease* your numerical quota and *increase* the time you take to do an exercise. Increased time spent in controlled, slower stretching is as important as the number of repetitions. For stubborn, tight muscles, hold each stretch between 30 seconds and a minute and cut your quota down to three repetitions.

Ground Rules for Physical Exercise

● Use preprogrammed skills as outlined in Chapter 7 in advance of exercise to insure relaxation during the exercise regimen.

● Use controlled breathing as described in Chapter 4 as your back-up if pain registers more sharply than expected.

● Always do warm-ups before tackling the actual regimen.

● Exercise twice each day—morning and evening. Follow each session with a warm, soothing shower or soak.

● If you're right-handed, begin each exercise with the left side of your body. If left-handed, begin on the right side.

The reason for this last ground rule is that the more you consciously involve *both* brain hemispheres in recovery activity, the more effective such activity is. When the *whole* brain is involved—and under forebrain control—you're in what might be described as a meditative state, one in which forebrain function (inhibitory of pain or negative feeling) is the rule. Since that's the whole point of programmed relaxation, beginning each exercise with the side of your body opposite the hand you write with reinforces the special nature of what you're doing.

Your Warm-up Routine

It's important to alert your body in advance of what you want it to do. That's what warming-up exercises are all about. Stretching, contracting and releasing muscles consciously prepares the body for greater exertion.

Do each of the following warm-ups *ten* times. It's best to do your warming up on the floor, but if your're bedridden, you can begin them while lying in bed. Warm-ups are always done slowly and never with jerking or bouncing motions.

1. Inhaling deeply through your nose, raise your arms slowly over your head. Exhale, returning your arms slowly to your sides.

2. Inhaling deeply, tense the muscles of your entire body slowly and clench your fists. Now exhale slowly, letting the body release all tension.

1.

2a.

2b.

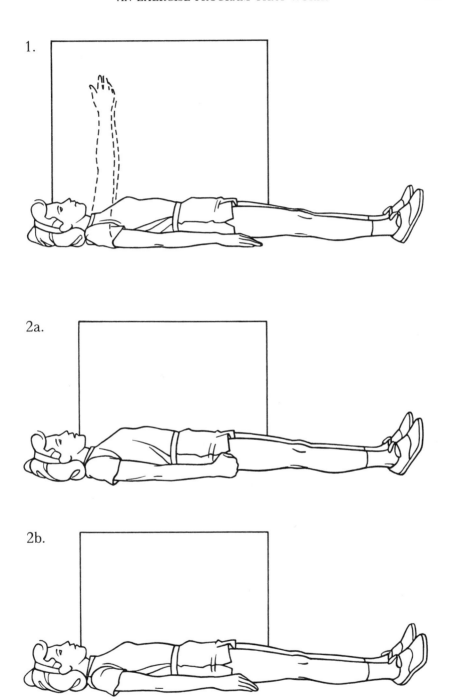

3. Bring your knees up to a flexed position, keeping your feet flat on the floor or mattress. Press down with your lower back. Raise your hips up as far as you comfortably can. Return to original position.

3a.

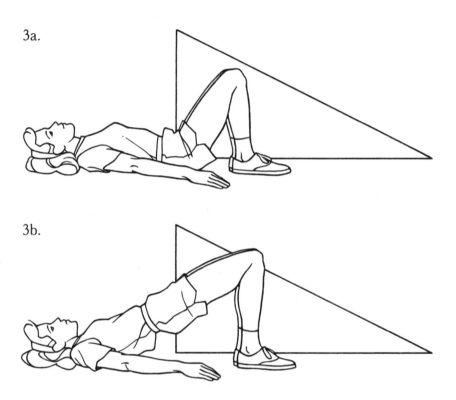

3b.

Toning Your Back and Abdominal Muscles

With warm-ups completed, you're ready to move into actually toning the muscle groups that provide the spinal column with stability and flexibility. Even bedridden people can do the first four of these exercises, but while all but the last one *can* be done in bed, do them on the floor as soon as possible.

The suggested quota is five repetitions of each exercise.

1. Lying on your back with legs straight, lift your leg as high as possible without bending your knee. Hold for five seconds before slowly lowering leg to floor. Do this five times. Repeat with your other leg.

1.

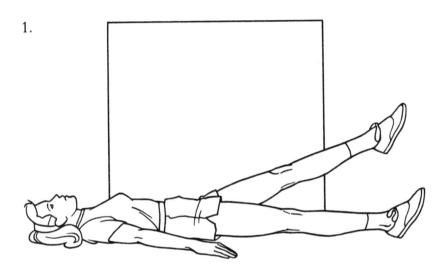

2. Still lying on your back, both legs extended, relax, then put your foot on the knee of your other leg. Slowly rotate your pelvis so that your first knee touches one side of the floor then the other. Do this five times, then reverse legs.

2a.

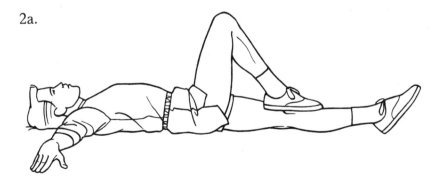

2b.

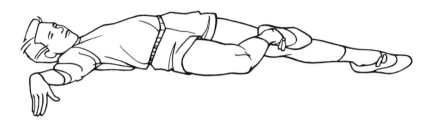

2c.

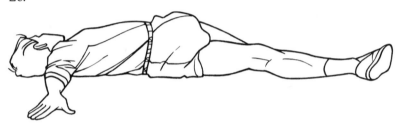

3.   Lie flat, knees up and together, feet flat on the floor (or
     mattress). You're going to be doing a modified sit-up, so

3.

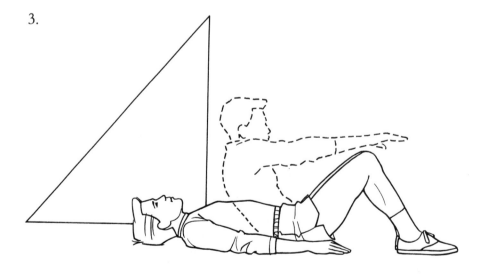

extend your arms, fingers toward knees, and *half* sit up. Your wrists should be over your knees. Lie back, keeping your legs in the flexed position, and repeat four more times.

4. Lying flat on your back, legs straight and knees together, lift your feet 12 inches into the air and hold them there for 10 seconds. Do not bend your knees, if possible. Then lower your legs slowly back to the original position.

4.

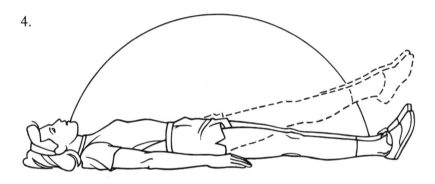

The remaining exercises may be too strenuous for Level One (Bedridden) people. However, bedridden people might try them cautiously and set goals that will make it possible to accomplish them gradually. These final two exercises are fine for Levels Two through Four.

5. Lying on your back, bring both knees up to the flex position, keeping your feet flat on the surface beneath you. Knees should be held together. Keep your back flat and swivel your

pelvis over to one side so that your knees touch the floor (or mattress), then swivel to the other side, knees touching the surface beneath you.

5a.

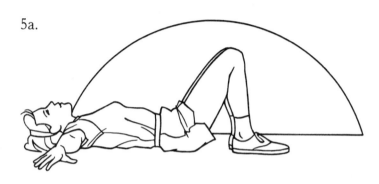

5b.

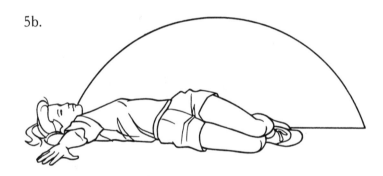

6. Stand straight behind a chair, holding its back with both hands. Bend your knees and squat—but just *halfway*. Hold for five seconds, then return to the starting position.

6.

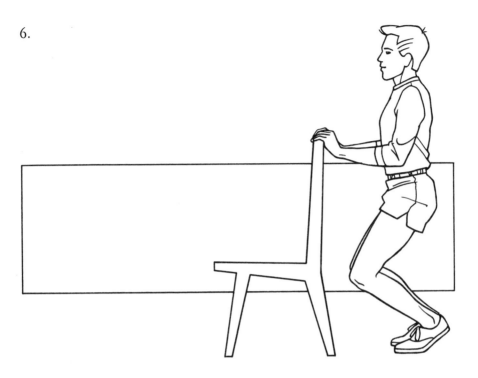

When you're able to perform all these exercises twice each day for a month, you should be ready for a new series of back and abdomen exercises.

Therapy in the Pool

Though mat exercise alone will begin to tone your muscles, we've also made water exercise a part of our program at Postural Therapeutics. The buoyancy of water relieves static stress, stimulates sensation in the skin and, if the water is 95 degrees or warmer, it helps relieve muscle tension.

If you have access to a pool, take advantage of it. The progress made by people who exercise in water is significant. If you don't have access to a private pool, check out the YMCA or YWCA facilities near you. Most "Y"s have a pool available to the public; so do many health spas and fitness centers. Some even offer water exercise therapy classes. The effort you'll be making is worth any inconvenience involved in getting to and from the pool, so if you're at Level Two or above, make the effort.

Water exercises are designed to provide maximum support for the body, depending on the muscles being toned. There are three types of exercise, based on how deep you stand in the water. You'll be doing all exercises close to the pool wall, so that if you should slip, it will be easy to resume a standing position.

The suggested quota is five repetitions of each full exercise. The following exercises are to be done in waist-deep water:

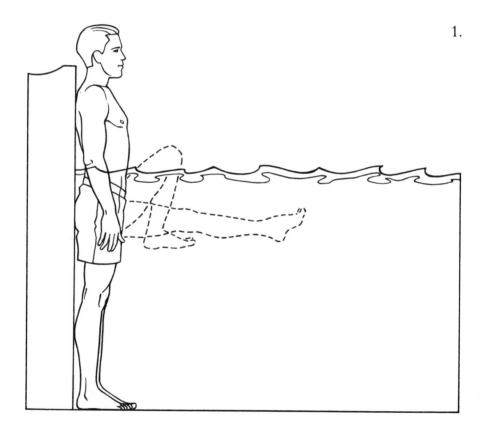

1.

1. Standing with your back against the pool wall, raise your knee up to your chest, then extend the leg, straightening it out completely. Return to the original position and do the same exercise with your other leg.

2. With your back still against the pool wall, raise your leg, clasping the shin with both arms, and pull your knee vigorously up to your chest. Return to standing position and do the same with your other leg.

2.

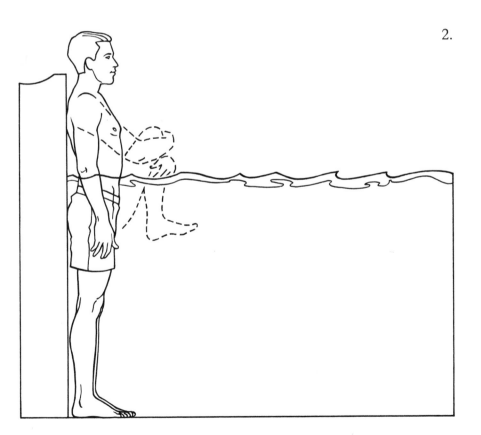

3. Raise your arm into the air. Keep it there and slowly bend
    to the opposite side as far as is comfortable. Return to the
    starting position, moving slowly and smoothly. Now do the
    same thing with your other arm.

3.

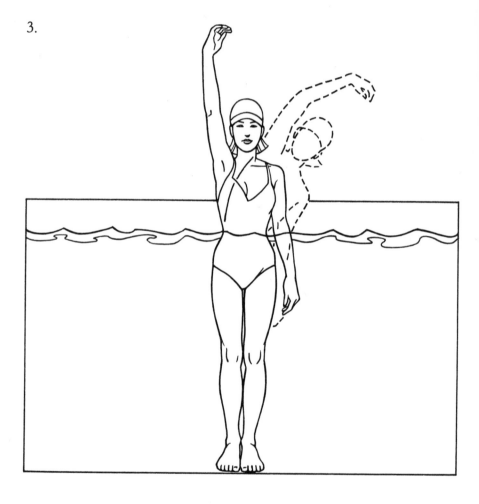

These exercises should be done in chest-deep water:

4. Bounce for ten seconds on one foot, using your hands for balance. Then bounce on your other foot.

4.

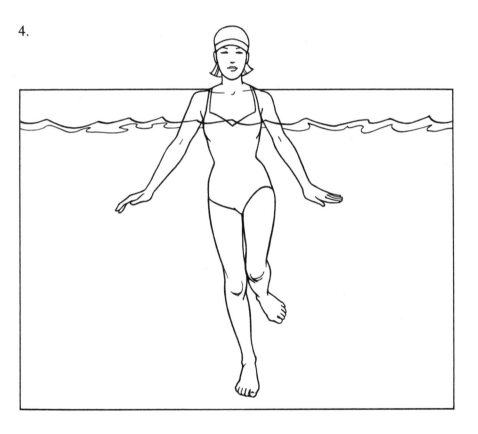

5. With your feet together, hands on hips, bounce on both feet and extend that bounce into a mild jump. Do *not* jump too high; that could create too much impact on the spine.

5.

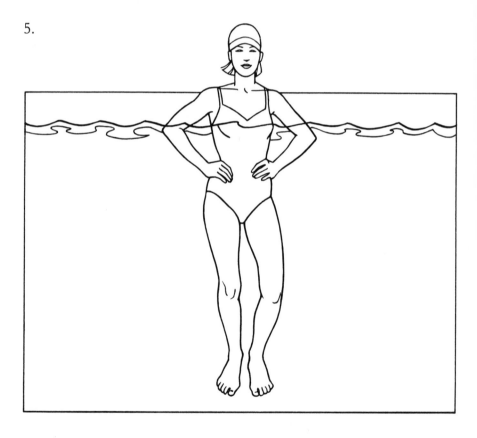

6. From a standing position, hands on hips, rise up on your toes—just as high as you can—then return to starting position. Accelerate as you do five repetitions.

6.

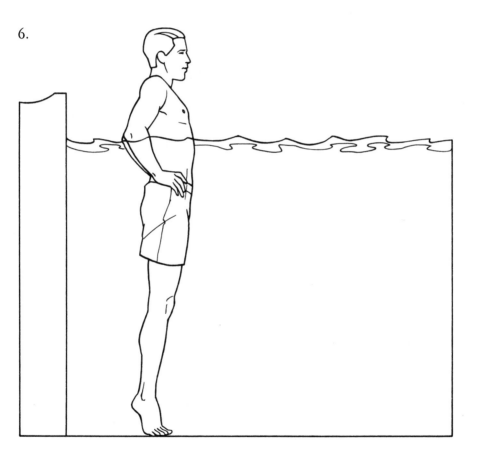

These exercises should be done in neck-deep water:

7. With your feet together and your back about 12 inches from
    the pool wall, twist to one side and touch the wall with both
    hands. Then twist the other way and touch the wall on your
    other side.

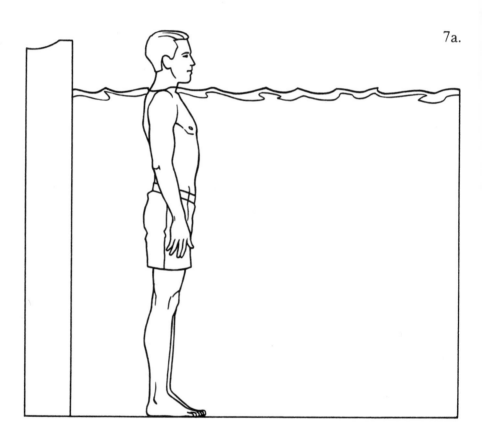

7a.

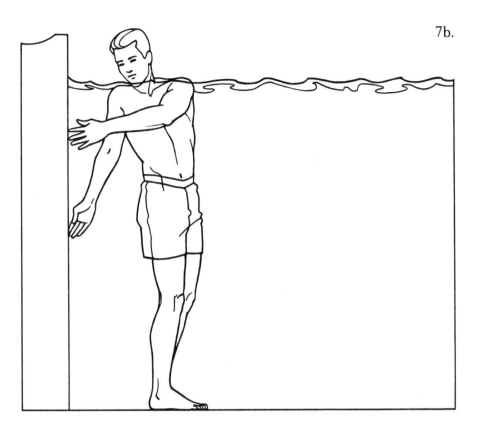

7b.

8. Reach back over your shoulders and hold on to the pool edge. Extend your legs straight out in front of you. Now swing your legs apart, then bring them together crossing one over the other. Swing your legs apart again, then bring them back together, this time crossing right over left.

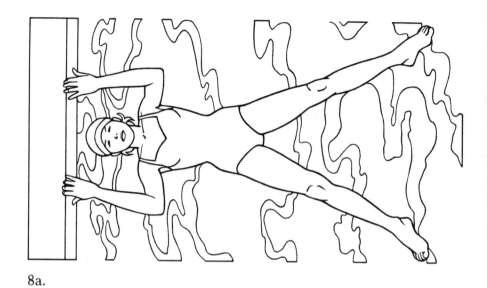

8a.

8b.

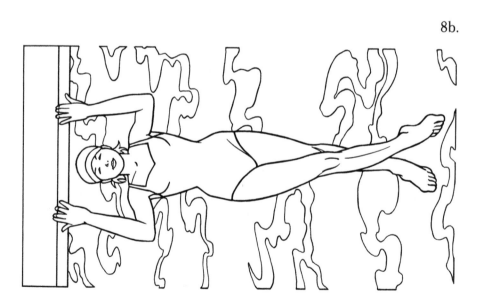

9. Again with your back against the wall, grasp the edge of the pool with both hands. Twist your hips to one side as far as you can, keeping your back flat to the pool's wall. Now return to the starting position and twist to the other side.

9a.

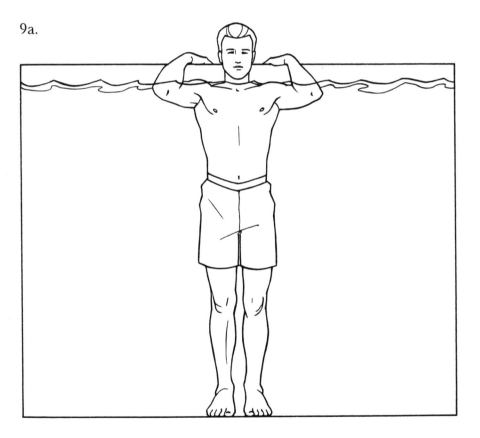

9b.

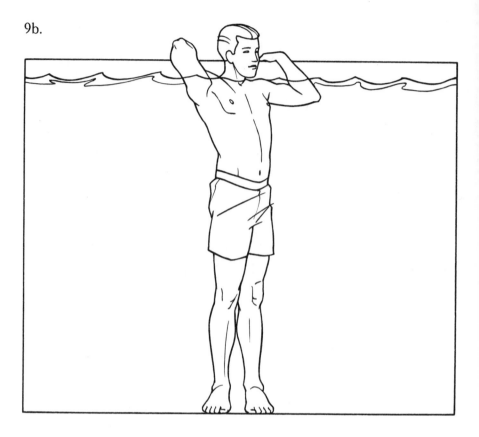

10. With the toes of your left foot touching the pool wall, your right foot behind you, take hold of the pool's edge and pull yourself forward, bending your left knee while the right straightens out behind you. Now bend the right knee and straighten the left. Reverse legs and repeat.

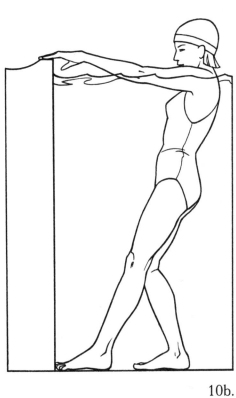

10a.

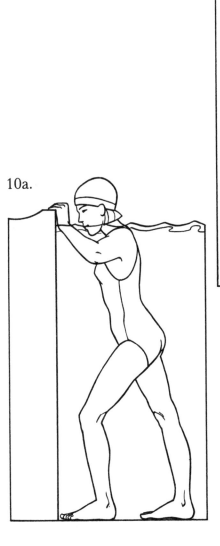

10b.

11.   Put both feet on the pool wall and take hold of the edge with
both hands. Pull your body forward by bending both knees,
then push back, straightening both legs.

11a.

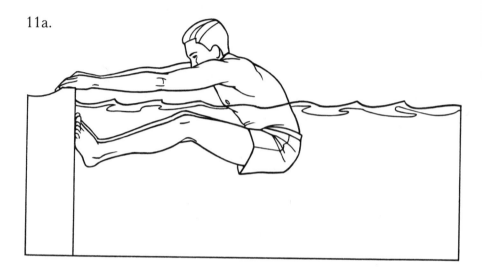

11b.

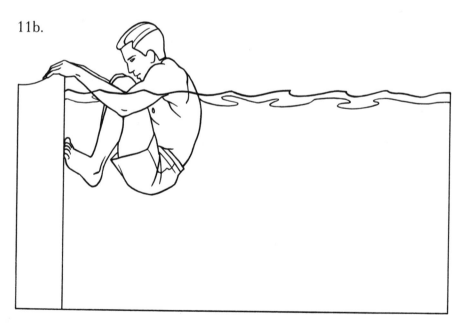

Make Everyday Tasks
Part of Your Exercise Program

Activity is exercise. Once you accept this simple reality, you can start using exercise to prepare yourself for specific on-the-job tasks. This is especially true if your acute attack began while you were bending, lifting or reaching while working. Such preparatory exercise is valuable for two reasons—it defuses fear of pain on an emotional level, and it provides assurance that you can indeed perform that activity with positive results.

People recovering from back problems are bound to attach undue anxiety to the physical actions that prompted their initial flare-up. That's why rehabilitation clinics across the country are developing unique programs that encourage back sufferers to actually perform those work-related physical activities while under clinical supervision. In a controlled setting, with appropriate staff standing by, such fears are dealt with directly.

Remember that conservative therapy, aggressively applied, operates on the assumption that the body can perform almost any task as long as pain is not the focus. Once you discover that you can bend or lift without increasing the pain, it becomes easier to bend or lift. Of course, reeducating yourself on how to lift and/or bend correctly makes a difference, too. But the *real* issue is personal motivation. Keep in mind that obliterating pain is not your ultimate goal; increasing activity is.

If going back to work is also one of your recovery goals, you can start building assurance that you can handle your job by rehearsing that job at home. Each element of your work involves specific activities such as sitting, standing, etc. Program these activities into your exercise regimen.

If your job requires you to be on your feet and moving around, start practicing now. Spend more time on your feet. Walk more and for longer distances. Figure out how long you're on your feet at work and set a recovery goal to stay on your feet for that length of time. When you've realized that goal, you're ready to return to work.

Relearning how to sit for long periods is another job-related skill for people in clerical or administrative work. One of my patients, an executive secretary named Joanne, found sitting very painful. She set up her bedroom as if it were an office and each day she sat and typed, actually working on projects. At first she typed for only a few minutes, but with each repetition, she made progress. When the pain became "too much," she got up and walked around, stretched, or rested for a few minutes in bed. Then she returned to her desk and her typing. Repetition of this practice finally made it possible for her to handle a time-frame equivalent to a full working day. Assured, she returned to work successfully.

Rehearsed repetition is an invaluable form of exercise, and whatever your work-related activities, you can make the same progress Joanne made if you'll think of those activities as exercise and build it into your recovery regimen.

Another example of this kind of controlled activity approach may help inspire recovering drivers to trust themselves on the road again. With the motor off, rehearse sitting behind the wheel of your car and go through the motions of driving. Then actually drive short distances for limited periods of time. When you feel ready, increase that time span, using controlled breathing to master any occasional painful twinges you might suffer.

Returning to work or an everyday lifestyle will involve specific physical activities. Identify those activities, think of them as exercise and make them part of your physical recovery program. When you realize that any consciously programmed and controlled activity counts as exercise, you can appreciate more fully that everything you do to get back into life's mainstream is helping you recover.

The more aggressively you move into living, the more support your body will provide. *If you can't do it the way you once did, find another way to do it.* Through visualization, preprogramming and controlled activity, you *can* find a way.

The same applies to sports, should that be one of your recovery goals. You know the specific motions involved in the sport you love. Turn those motions into physical exercise and rehearse them as a part of your recovery regimen. The more you practice them, the easier they'll become. Don't make the mistake of assuming you can just start playing again. Prepare yourself, removing as many variables as possible from your reentry into active sports. And don't take on a sport that's beyond your ability or condition.

Exercising on the Job

Once you return to work, your muscles need even more reinforcement toning. The stress and strain of being back in the workplace is likely to affect you by threatening destructive stress. Take a break in your work schedule to do the following exercises. As consciously controlled activity combined with physical exercise, they'll program relaxation to break the cycle of destructive stress as well as tone your muscles.

You can do these exercises in the lunchroom, employee lounge, at your workbench or in your office. All you need is a chair and a solid desk or worktable.

If you're concerned about what onlookers may think, tell them exactly what you're doing and why it's important. Your example may be inspiring. I know of several situations where recovering back sufferers have motivated co-workers to the point where they turned coffee breaks into short exercise sessions.

These exercises are also ideal for people who've never had an acute attack. They're superb preventive exercises, especially for "weekend warriors" who sit at desks all week and then overexert themselves on weekends playing racquetball, volleyball, football and other sports that require a lot of physical stamina and strength.

On-the-Job Warm-ups

As with any exercise program, begin with warm-ups to alert the body and stretch key muscle groups. Most Level Three people and all Level Fours can use both the warm-ups and the exercises in this section. Again I want to emphasize, however, that stretching exercises must be done *slowly* and with complete mental control.

Even if you've reached Level Three or Four—or are using these exercises as preventive therapy, don't "bounce" or "force" stretching activity. I frequently see people "warming up" for a sport by jumping and bouncing all over the place; that's a very good way to strain a muscle. Consciously controlled *slow* stretching of the muscles is what you're aiming for, not a feeling of physical stress. Stress equals tension, and tension equals problems. So do these warm-ups slowly, evenly; control each beginning, middle and end. Use controlled breathing before and after each of them.

1. Sitting in a chair, arms to your sides, bend forward until your chest and thighs touch. Now extend your arms ahead of your knees. Keep them straight and hold that stretch for ten seconds. Repeat three times.

1.

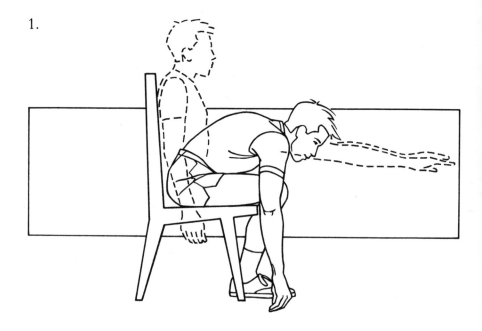

2.   Still in your chair with feet flat on the floor and hands in your
     lap, bend as far as you can to the left, keeping your spine
     parallel to the back of the chair. Hold for ten seconds. Do the
     same to the right. Repeat both left/right maneuvers three
     times.

3.   Stand behind a table or desk that won't slide under your
     weight. You'll be supporting yourself with your hands. With
     arms straight and extended, palms flat on the table, move
     back far enough so your body makes something like a
     45-degree angle to the floor. You'll feel your calf and thigh
     muscles stretch. Once in position, hold for ten seconds.
     Return to a standing position and repeat three times.

2.

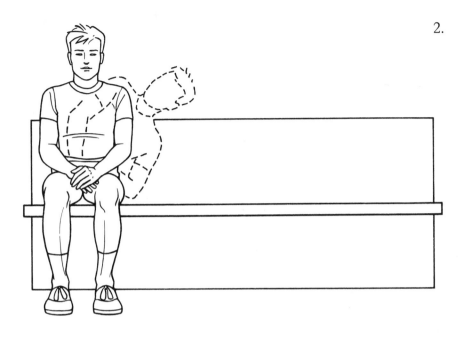

3.

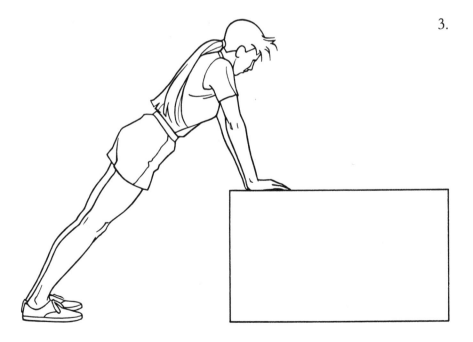

Your On-the-Job Exercise Program

With your warm-ups complete, you're ready for the actual exercises. As you read them, you're likely to think, what a piece of cake. But believe me, they're not that easy for people recovering from back problems. What's more, they involve key muscle groups that are rarely exercised consciously in this manner. That's why these exercises are so useful.

As with all exercise, stay in conscious control and use controlled breathing before and after. These exercises are to be done *slowly* to increase the benefits of controlled stretching.

1. Sit in your chair with your back straight and both feet on the floor. Lift one knee toward your nose as far as you can. Return to the original position. Now do the same with your other knee. Repeat the exercise, only this time bend slightly forward. Repeat eight times. As it gets easier, straighten your back and keep it straight.

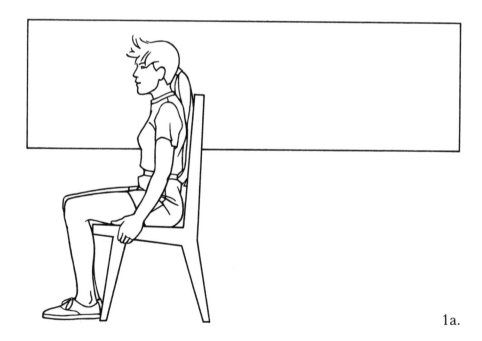

1a.

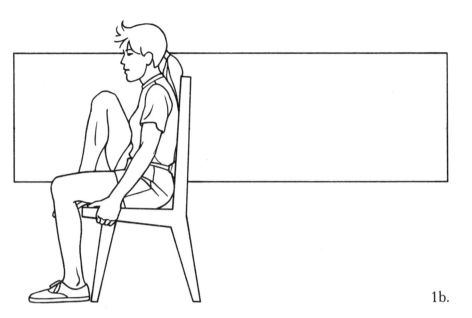

1b.

2.   While sitting straight, cross one knee over the other. Return your foot to the floor. Alternate legs. As you grow stronger

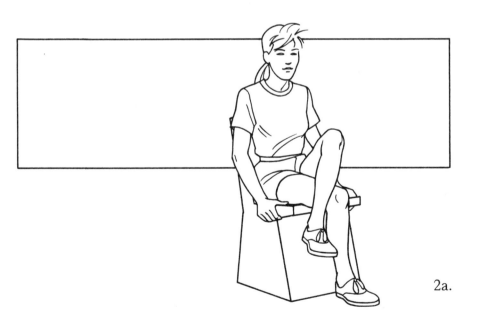

2a.

and more limber, lean back on the chair and lift your knees
higher and higher as you do this exercise. Eight crosses for
each leg equals one set.

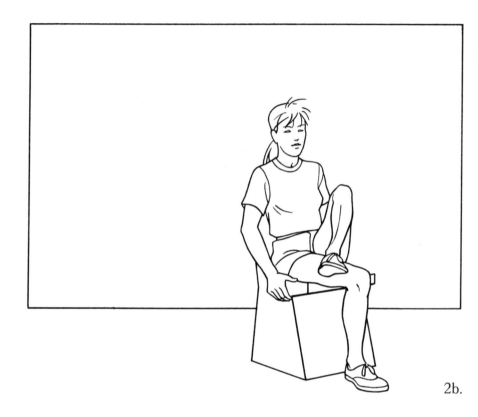

2b.

3. Sit straight, feet flat on the floor, holding the chair arms
   firmly. *Slowly* turn, looking to one side as far as is comfortable. Now repeat to the other side. Never jerk or make
   sudden sharp movements. Use the chair arms to keep from
   slumping. Do eight twists to each side.

3.

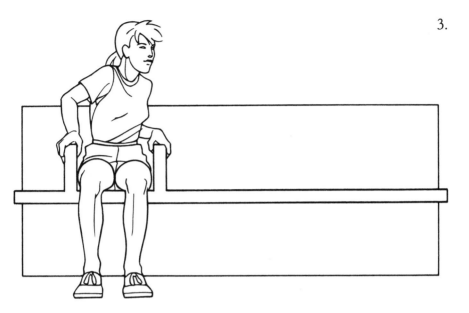

4. Take off your shoes for the next two exercises. Sit with your feet about 12 inches apart. Heels on the floor, turn both feet inward, then outward. Repeat 20 times.

4.

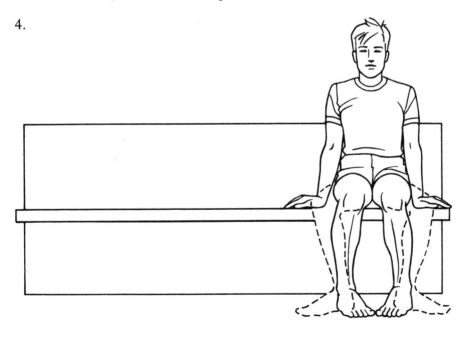

5.   Put your knees and ankles together. Your heels should be slightly under the chair, ankles bent. Raise your heels, keeping the ball of the foot and toes on the floor, then lower your heels again. Repeat 20 times.

5.

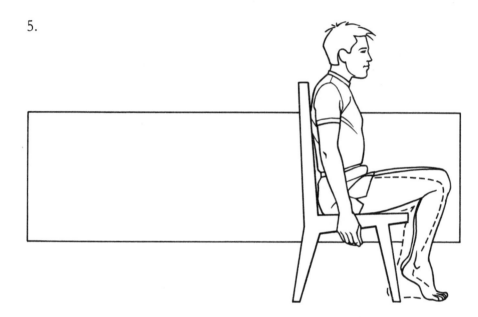

6.   Sit in a chair, grasp the arms firmly and lift your torso slowly, keeping your feet flat on the floor. Slowly lower yourself back into a sitting position. Repeat eight times.

NOTE: If your back tells you this one is too difficult right now, begin by pushing up from the chair *seat*—palms flat on the seat, arms straight. As soon as you can do so comfortably, graduate to using the chair's arms. And as soon as possible, raise your feet from the floor at the same time you lift your torso.

7.   Stand facing your chair. Take hold of its arms and place one foot on the chair seat. Return your foot to the floor. Repeat with your other foot. Start with 10 repetitions and work up to 40.

6.

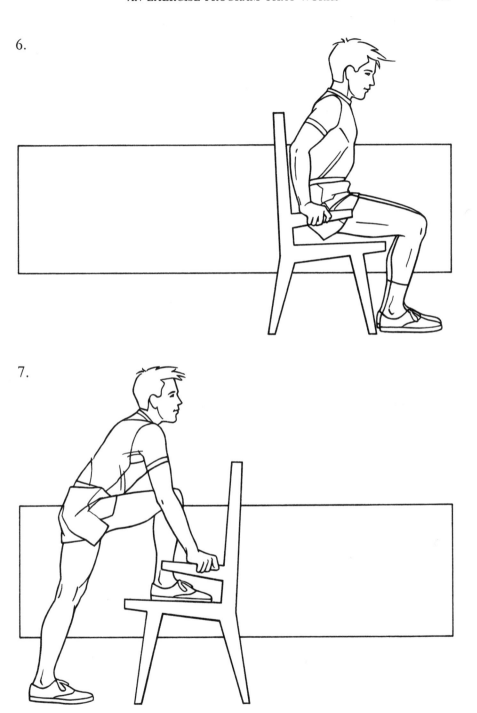

7.

8. Use a desk, table or chair for support. Slowly lower yourself
    into a half-knee bend. Repeat five times.

8.

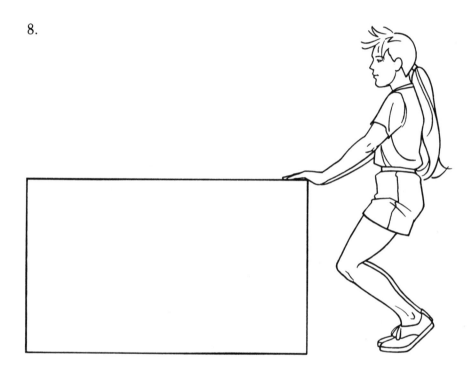

9. Stand away from a desk or table that can't slide under your
    weight. Place both hands on the table and lower your chest
    toward its surface. Go as slowly as you can. Be far enough
    away that your back is straight and your feet are flat on the
    floor. Always tighten your abdominals to support your
    lumbar area while you do this exercise. When you've reached
    your comfort limit, return to the first position. Repeat five

9a.

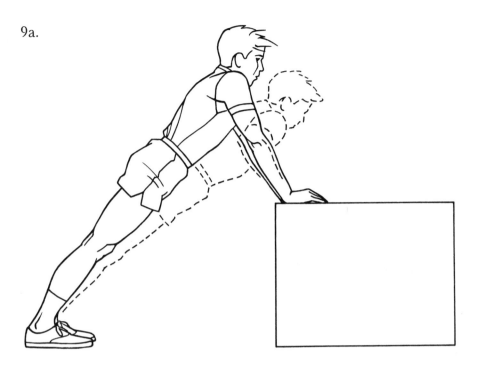

times. As your Level of Activity increases and your range of motion improves, transfer from a table top to a chair, then to a low sturdy box, and finally to the floor.

9b.

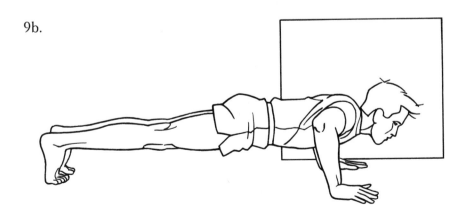

Setting Exercise Goals

Goals set for us by others are rarely achieved. That's why I'm simply suggesting a pattern of exercise. If it sounds viable to you, choose to make this pattern your own. But set your own goals, set your own quotas, then go to work achieving them.

For those of you who are working your way up from Level One or Two, accept the fact that there may be discomfort, or even pain, as you begin your physical exercise recovery program. Expect it, then bypass it; put your full attention on *controlling* this activity. Once you start, keep going—and remember, half-effort doesn't produce half-results; it produces *no* results.

Another reminder: Note your physical exercise goals and quotas in your recovery journal. Once a week, evaluate your progress in attaining these goals and quotas. Once you've fulfilled them, set new quotas and goals. Be sure to write down all perceived improvements and to reward yourself for each attainment; celebrate your progress.

Finally, understand and accept that getting better is a full-time job—a vocation. Continued, controlled regular exercise must become a way of life; it's the only hopeful way to insure a *future* life free from the pain of a bad back.

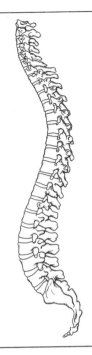

Recovery and Making Love

The following case history is intimate in nature, and I tell it only with the express permission of the patient involved. Naturally, I won't use her real name.

Candace first came to me after enduring two years of chronic lower back pain—pain for which no clear clinical cause could be found. Even as one of the walking wounded, she retained the vestiges of what must have been remarkable beauty. But she didn't seem to care how she looked; like so many chronic sufferers, nothing but her pain was real to her anymore.

Candace had been raised by religious parents, people who found it impossible to discuss with her what were then known as "the facts of life." She was a virgin when she married Stephan, and very innocent for her age. Sexual intercourse was painful at first, but that passed. Unfortunately, she remembered the pain, and while she never refused her husband, she never encouraged him either. Later Stephan would tell me that he too was sexually innocent when they married. While he'd been an eager partner, he hadn't been a patient one.

Candace suffered an acute back attack shortly after she and Stephan returned from their honeymoon. She had been vacuuming and bent over to turn off the machine. Blinding pain struck her lower back. Unable to straighten up, she lay down on the floor until the initial spasm passed. Finally she managed to crawl to the couch, which is where she stayed until Stephan found her when he returned from work. He helped her into bed, where she remained for the next two days.

From that day until she came to me, Candace had been through the gamut of doctors and treatments, but her pain remained almost constant. During those two years, she had tried to maintain the physical side of her marriage, but each sexual encounter was agonizing. Just the weight of Stephan's body on hers made her gasp with pain, but when he suggested positions other than the one she considered normal, she reacted with moral indignation. Candace could no longer conceal the revulsion she felt when her husband turned to her in the night. Each encounter ended with her in tears. Stephan finally moved into the guest bedroom.

Telling me this, she wept bitterly. "Now he *never* touches me, not even to kiss me goodnight."

"Do you want him to touch you?"

"Of course! At least until he begins to take me in his arms. Then I'm so afraid of the pain, I turn away."

I asked Candace what it was she thought I could do for her that other doctors had been unable to accomplish.

"You're a surgeon," she snapped. "Operate!"

I explained that surgery was a last resort, and if she wanted to become a patient of mine, we would have to begin by scheduling a battery of tests. Convinced that I would find something her previous doctors hadn't, she agreed to enter the hospital.

Candace's pain was very real, but my clinical findings echoed the many others in her medical records. Surgery was not indicated, I told her, and if performed would probably only worsen her situation. As she had many times before, she succumbed to hysteria. If she couldn't become "a whole woman" again, her husband would surely leave her. Without him, life would have no meaning.

Every doctor she'd seen had told her to exercise, and she considered it standard jargon. It was too pat an answer, and she knew in her heart it wouldn't work. As far as biofeedback training was concerned, it wasn't for her. If prayer didn't work, nothing would.

I didn't see Candace for over a month. By the time she came into my office again, she was haggard with defeat. Her husband had accused her of using her back as an excuse not to make love and, after a terrible row, he had walked out on her. The pain of losing him was even greater than the pain she felt in her body. Now she was so desperate that she would do anything to save her marriage. I could see that at last she had the motivation to get well. All she needed now was to make the mental turnaround.

I again asked her to consider a rehabilitation clinic. There she could begin a program of therapeutic exercise and have an opportunity to interact with other back and neck patients. She would also receive practical instruction in posture, body mechanics, diet and pain alleviation. At the very least, the relaxation skills she learned might help relieve her emotional pain. The clinic also offered psychological counseling that would help her understand and master her Pain Behavior.

It wasn't her pain that drove her husband away, I explained, it was her Pain Behavior. She asked me to elaborate, and for the first time I saw Candace smile (if somewhat bitterly) as she acknowledged that she had been practicing not only Pain Behavior but Pain Manipulation as well.

With my prescription, she entered into a program at a rehabilitation clinic and began a regimen of mat and pool exercise tailored to her needs. With biofeedback training, she learned to maintain relaxation in the face of pain, and each time we talked, I could see her attitude improving. Eight months later, she was the picture of radiance, beautifully groomed and dressed. Her face glowed when she proudly told me she and her husband were together again—and making love.

"Not just having sex," she said, "but making love." The distinction seemed important to her, and it was. She had based her whole recovery program on that distinction, and this is what she'd done:

One day, after her first week at the rehab clinic, Candace went home, stripped and stood in front of a full-length mirror. Her body, conforming to pain, had lost its erect posture, much of its shape and all of its muscle tone. Remembering our conversation on Pain Behavior, she realized she'd not only let her appearance go, she'd become a complaining whiner. No wonder Stephan had left. Who'd want to live with—much less make love to—a whimpering, negative woman who only talked pain and medical case history? How could he even have wanted sex with someone whose mind was dulled by medication, whose body had become desensitized to anything but pain?

From that day on, she willed herself to stay out of bed for longer periods of time. Gritting her teeth, she continued her morning critique at the mirror.

Eating had become a way to satisfy her feelings of loneliness and isolation. Not only was her muscle tone bad, she was 20 pounds overweight.

At the rehab clinic, she found books relating to muscle composition and discovered that green leafy vegetables, yellow vegetables and certain dairy products such as yogurt and buttermilk seemed beneficial for conditions like hers. So did organ meats such as liver. Fresh citrus provided a natural source of Vitamin C. Fish would provide other dietary advantages. She also read that reducing intake of refined sugar and flour would hasten weight loss. For a long time she'd been relying on frozen foods, canned goods and fast-food chain stores—anything that didn't involve standing for long periods of time to prepare and/or cook.

Deciding "fresh was best," Candace made daily grocery shopping one of her goals. She lived near a major supermarket, and she began walking there and back. Success convinced her that she could extend her limits, so she increased that journey to a farmer's market four full blocks beyond the supermarket. None of this exercise was free from pain, but pain had been her excuse before and she refused to give way again to that justification.

After several weeks, the mirror was telling her a different story. Her posture was better—her body was reshaping. Daily exercise at home and three weekly trips to the clinic had resulted in visible progress. Her muscle tone was returning. She then set the most important goal of her life. She wanted her husband back, but she couldn't expect him to live a celibate life. She wanted to share her body with the man she loved; it was the greatest symbol of their oneness. But she had never enjoyed sex and had finally come to equate it with pain. If she really wanted her marriage to work, she must make a commitment that pain wouldn't stand in her way. She made having sex—and enjoying it—her ultimate goal.

This commitment had two aspects. Her physical activity level must increase. And mentally, she'd have to change her attitudes about sex, which meant learning more than she'd known before marriage. To increase her physical abilities, Candace augmented her trips to the clinic. Now she was going five times a week with a Saturday trip to a beauty salon thrown in for good measure. To secure the kind of education she needed to expand her awareness about sex and sexual expression, she read the works of Masters and Johnson. She learned that sexual dysfunction between couples was often based on a lack of intimacy and ignorance of the sensuous nature of their bodies. She learned of the need to sensualize the act of love, to create experiences that were new and could resensitize her body.

When the mirror reflected a figure she was proud of, and her body told her it could sustain the activity planned, Candace telephoned Stephan. It amused her that at first he didn't recognize her voice; it wasn't the whining, complaining tone he'd become so used to. He was cautious about making a date; the memory of two years of listening to stories about pain and medical history, and the thought of more of the same, was hardly his idea of a good time. She assured him neither subject was on the agenda. Surprised by her upbeat attitude, he agreed to see her.

They met at a restaurant a few blocks from her home. Candace looked lovely and sat through a long meal, keeping the conversation on generalities. Not one word about pain passed her lips. By the end of the meal, Stephan was seeing her with new eyes. Curious, he asked what she'd been doing to create such a dramatic change. She briefly reviewed her regimen at the clinic, but told him that *what* she was doing was secondary to *why* she was doing it. She wanted him back, she wanted his love again. Completely honest, she admitted that physical love wasn't in their immediate future but, she explained, she was working on it.

Stephan balked at the thought of moving back in with Candace, but agreed to see her whenever she wanted and assured her that she had his support. Motivated by thoughts of reconciliation, Candace worked even harder to recover.

Combining the calm from her biofeedback and relaxation training with the visualization process she learned at the clinic, she put aside a special time every day when she could relax, close her eyes and visualize what she wanted to share with the man she loved.

When she felt ready, Candace invited Stephan over for dinner. She set the stage beautifully; the table was decorated with candles and flowers. Dinner was simple, but she'd taken the time and energy to prepare it from scratch, reminding herself that added time spent standing and moving about the kitchen was yet another form of exercise. The stress of her expectations increased her pain awareness, but she focused on her breathing patterns to relax and played music that was part of her self-created biofeedback pain-monitoring pattern.

He marvelled at her progress and told her she seemed very much her old self again. No, Candace corrected, she was her *new* self, a self in the process of being created from the ground up. For the first time, they communicated on a mature level. She asked if he wanted to save their marriage. He assured her he still loved her, but needed a marriage that was fulfilling on every level—including the physical. Candace told him that was what she wanted, too, but physically, it would be some time before she could engage in full sexual intercourse. In the meantime, they could both learn something about the sensual aspects of lovemaking. She explained the visualization process and told him what she had visualized for them to do that night.

Surprised to hear her speak so candidly about sex, Stephan told her that playing sex games would be difficult without those games culminating in intercourse, but he was so delighted with the "new" Candace that he'd agree to anything.

Some of the movements involved in disrobing still caused Candace pain; things would go more smoothly if he did the work and she kept centered on relaxation. He removed his own clothing, then hers, just as she'd visualized. Then she led him into the bathroom, where she filled the tub with steaming water and a foaming, jasmine-scented bath oil. Together they relaxed in the perfumed warmth, lightly caressing, exploring and enjoying each other's body. Neither of them wanted the session to end, but finally the exertion took its toll and Candace called a halt before pain overwhelmed pleasure.

The next step in her plan was sensuous massage. Before their next date, she stretch-tested muscles that would be involved in giving a massage. Then she employed her relaxation and visualization techniques again and when the time was right, invited her husband over again.

Both nude, they took turns massaging each other in an atmosphere of candlelight, roses and warm, scented oil. Candace was first to be massaged; she knew she'd find added reserves of energy for the relaxation that would bring. His touch was smooth, sensuous and slow. To her surprise, Candace realized that the hollow of her throat and her upper arms were erogenous zones; so were her feet and calves. Although she knew she wasn't yet ready for intercourse, for the first time she yearned for the act of sex. Living out the dream she'd visualized, stronger sensations than pain dulled her discomfort.

When Stephan's turn came, Candace discovered that touching him was as erotic as being touched by him. Nothing in her upbringing or his suggested that it was proper for a woman to touch a man as a man touched a woman, and the strangeness of this role reversal was stimulating to them both. As the massage progressed, both realized they were letting go of conditioned attitudes and expectations. Warm, soothing strokes of flesh that had never before been touched in foreplay were more arousing than traditional foreplay had ever been.

As she massaged his body, Candace spoke quietly about the body's energy, flowing, moving, radiating, just as the clinic's masseuse talked about to her. And like the masseuse, she spoke of the body as a vital living organism that functioned best when it was relaxed, when its energy was balanced, free from stress and strain. What they were sharing in massage was a blending of those energies, Candace told Stephan—a kind of synthesis in sharing because they loved each other.

After the massage, they lay together on her bed. He found himself communicating more freely than ever before, as if their exchange of loving touch had brought a new acceptance. Old taboos began to dissolve. They'd never discussed his work-related problems in the past, but suddenly he was telling her about his fears and conflicts on the job. And the more they talked, the more they opened up. He told Candace how inadequate he'd felt at home during her two years of chronic pain; how guilty for not being able to help her get better. It was that guilt, he confessed, that finally drove him away—not her inability to have sex.

The intimacy of his confession amazed and freed them both. Holding hands, they lay in darkness, satisfied to be touching and together. After all, there is nothing more seductive than a sense of complete freedom and openness, and that was what they knew they now shared—equality and honesty.

Mutual massage sessions continued for another two weeks; so did the intimate conversations afterward. This growing intimacy, both physical and emotional, convinced Candace that it was time to attempt the first stage of sexual involvement. Her loving touch became purposefully sensual. Lying next to him after massage, she fondled and caressed his sexual organs, totally clearing her mind of past conditioning that told her such fondling was taboo for a woman. If this was the safest way to bring her husband to climax without causing herself discomfort, it served a valuable purpose. And when he returned her loving touch in kind, with the same sense of newness and discovery, Candace began to experience her own body in a different and enormously exciting fashion.

Between two people who love each other, sex in any form can and should be a joy. What Candace and her husband began to realize was that the heart had been missing in their relationship. Certainly their love had not extended fully into sex. For both, the act had been just that—an act in which climax meant more than caring. Now caring was preeminent. Now every touch of their bodies brought a desire for even deeper intimacy.

After orgasm, they lay quietly beside each other, grateful for the sharing that brought them so much closer in spirit as well as feeling. Candace let the wonderful afterglow spread throughout her body, centering it like warmth in the tense back muscles that plagued her still. That healing warmth, the warmth of expressed love, seemed more nurturing than even the relaxation created by her biofeedback training.

Mutual masturbation brought them closer and closer over the weeks that followed. After orgasm they verbalized their dreams, quietly discussing their fears and problems. Naturally one of the topics was the next phase of their physical intimacy. For both, oral sex had been a taboo; their upbringing had taught them that the idea of touching sexual organs with the mouth was wrong. Still, both had experienced such a sense of oneness on so many levels during this period that it seemed a natural step in the evolution of their newfound intimacy.

Besides, the positions for oral sex need put little (if any) strain upon the back. This time *he* was the first to undertake the exploration. The unfamiliar intimate sensations excited by his tongue were as amazing as the sense of ecstasy she felt. Reciprocating wasn't easy the first time. She had him stand beside the bed where she sat in relative comfort, careful to control the motions and degree of penetration. Making love orally was more difficult physically for her than for him at first, but practice brought proficiency.

This was the turning point in their relationship. I don't mean to imply that oral sex is the key to lifelong companionship—nor was Candace confused about that issue. The point is that the very nature of what she and her husband were creating on a physical level partook of such honesty, respect and caring that it was inevitable they would reconcile. They'd become best friends; there was intimacy on every level they shared.

Neither could bear the thought of losing that intimacy. The day he moved back into their old apartment, there was no question about permanence. Everything had been discussed, everything was clear. Clearest of all was Candace's demonstration that pain need never again be the problem that pushed them apart. It had in fact been the thing that brought them together. Her mastery of self set her husband the best possible example of self-direction and self-control.

From Candace he learned to handle stress more effectively. From sharing their bodies in a new context of intimacy, he learned to care for and respect those bodies more completely. With the mystery removed about their bodies, it was easier to understand the mysteries of their minds—the conditioning and attitudes toward self that were real problems in their (and anyone's) relationship. Once acknowledged, these problems were halfway to being solved.

Most important of all, it was a joy to be together. On the day of his return home—some three months after their first "date"—they had what they used to think of as their "normal" sex. Lying on their sides, her back to him, his kisses on her neck and shoulders, fitting together like two spoons, Candace's husband entered her body. This position guaranteed the most comfort for her since less pressure was focused on her back. Best of all, in this position they could remain joined after orgasm, fully sharing that wonderful sense of warmth and oneness—and drift off to sleep embracing.

The Revolving Reward process of this experience increased Candace's motivation even more. Daily exercise had been the rule, but from that moment she worked even harder in order to achieve more. Sex had been the motivator. For Candace, mastering her pain permitted her to overcome *all* life's obstacles. In her case, love became the healer.

Candace's courage in taking the initiative in such a sensitive area as sexual expression is unparalled in my experience. Her upbringing left her with moralistic taboos that affected her image of what making love should and shouldn't be. Like all of us, Candace had more to overcome than a back problem.

If your upbringing has conditioned you to believe that only certain acts or positions are acceptable—or that it's wrong to enjoy sex—you probably had a problem with sex before your acute attack or chronic condition. When pain enters the picture, whatever problems you had will multiply. Pain provides us with the perfect excuse not to do what we don't *want* to do. It becomes our justification. Should you elect to reactivate sexual expression during recovery without changing your attitudes, you'll face major stumbling blocks along the way.

The primary problem is not the pain; that's a given. The primary problem is how you feel about having sex. If, like Candace, it's important to you, you'll find a way to make love again. If your attitudes toward sex—or toward your sexual partner—are still problems, however, Pain Behavior is likely to continue in that area.

As a physician, I feel that back sufferers need never eliminate sex from a loving relationship. Physically, there are always alternative ways of achieving that all-important sense of intimacy which can, of itself, be so healing. Even Level One or Two recoverers can at least achieve some degree of sexual satisfaction with their partners. Of course, for the time being, their approach to making love will be altered, but some physical expression of that love need never be lost.

Candace reeducated both mind and body to achieve her goal. She rebuilt the whole relationship, step by step, and put love back into her life. Her reward was an intimacy she'd never known before. That intimacy was worth all the struggle, all the pain and exertion needed to make it possible. If sex was a problem area for you prior to your pain, consider what she accomplished and *how* she accomplished it. Applying that example, or at least part of it, could reestablish a truly loving relationship in your life.

I'm a surgeon, not a psychiatrist or sexologist. As much as possible, I stick to the facts. But the awareness of supportive love is such a boost to physical recovery that I feel compelled to share some of my thinking with you when it comes to making love. If this helps you make the mental turnaround in the most intimate relationship of your life, I'll feel I've been of service.

As far as your beliefs and attitudes about sex go, you'll need to examine them amid the inner silence of your mental "sand dune." But in addition to any such problems you need to address, there is a specific physical condition that relates to chronic suffering and/or spinal surgery. This physical condition is very real.

Surgery, Prolonged Pain and Erogenous Sensation

When a disc herniates, it puts pressure on surrounding nerves. In the lower spine, many of these nerves control sensation not only in the bladder and bowel, but in the sexual organs and adjacent erogenous zones, including thighs and buttocks. Surgical intervention sometimes causes desensitization. Because this dulling of sense response isn't as apparent as the pain caused by a slipped disc, people aren't always clearly aware that such desensitization has taken place.

The same is often true as the result of chronic suffering. People who live on Level One or Two are immersed in almost constant pain. During such prolonged agony, sexual thoughts and images are usually consciously repressed. In the process, we're unconsciously giving our brain a command that sex is not to be desired. Such a mindset further desensitizes our bodies, and desensitization can persist well into recovery—especially if we do nothing to turn our attitudes around and refocus on making love as something we really want to do.

Without such a mental turnaround, instead of expecting pleasure from sex, we expect pain; and psycho-physiological pain is what we get. Our fear of pain, as real as pain itself, reinforces the belief that sex is denied us by our bodies. Rather than risk finding out whether it really is or not, many men and women become impotent or frigid. "It hurts so much I don't *want* to do it" transforms into "It hurts so much I *can't* do it."

And yet the allure of sex, the romance of being wanted, can be the very motivation that inspires progress. If, like Candace, you want love, you'll find a way to make love, one step at a time. Remember, orgasm should never be the primary goal. The primary goal should be to resensitize your body so that you can enjoy whatever level of sexual activity is possible. And should you still shy away from the idea of sex due to fear of pain, let me give you some reasons why physical intimacy can aid your recovery process.

Sex Is Great for Your Back

If all the world's orthopedic specialists convened to formulate the best single exercise for releasing muscular constriction, toning back muscles and relaxing the nervous system, making love would be that exercise. It accomplishes all the above and more.

Sex Is Not a Boring Form of Exercise

Stretching, jogging, mat and pool exercise can all become tedious. But there are so many ways to make love that there's always a process of discovery. Plus, you're not exercising alone. With a partner, you're much more likely to stick with an exercise regimen. Progress is apparent in the increased quality and activity of sex.

Orgasm Is the Best Muscle Relaxant Around

Orgasm has a profound effect on the entire body. Scientifically, it has been demonstrated that orgasm has ten times the effect of Valium. In addition, the deep inhalations and exhalations following the orgasm itself continue the relaxation process of muscles and nerves. For back sufferers, the ten minutes following a sexual climax can be a healing luxury not to be denied.

Only Touch Is a Stronger Sensation Than Pain
Within the nervous system, only touch has priority over pain. Being held calms the crying infant; we embrace in sympathy or love. Being touched or stroked is soothing; we do it naturally. Only the most intense pain is given priority over touch. In sex, the touching sensation is internal as well as external, increasing the intensity of the sensation.

This last point is extremely important when it comes to reeducating a pain-wracked body in preparation for making love. Such bodies may be physically out of touch with sensation except in terms of pain. It's only through the choice to want physical love that the body is alerted to respond anew. And yet there is another choice to be made as well: More significant than to want physical love is the desire to *enjoy* it.

The Need to Sensualize Sex

Any recovery takes place in stages. In making love, the first priority is rediscovering sensation. Candace's story outlines the basic pattern. With orgasm *not* the object, she found ways to share her body with the man she loved. More than touch was involved; she planned the stimulation of every sense input. The savor of the meal she'd prepared, the candlelight, the aroma of sweet-smelling bath water, special music to charm the ear—all these were part of her resensualization process. Later came the loving touch and the smooth sensation of warm oil. And with massage, Candace became aware that she had erogenous zones other than the expected ones.

Candace and Stephan were having *fun*. They were doing new things in new ways; sharing new experiences, experiences unique in their lives. This is the stuff romance is made of, the delight of courtship renewed. Beyond all else, they were becoming intimate, at one with each other. And not just in terms of sex; discovering their sensuous side gave them the freedom to rediscover an open line of communication on any subject. Together, they had discovered a way to handle the pain of life which both had endured alone.

Anyone in a committed relationship can profit from their example, for without a commitment to consciously sensualize the experience of physical love, sex becomes commonplace. When it does, all other mutual areas of activity suffer. Being taken for granted is extremely painful, especially when it relates to the most intimate act two people can share. It reads as genuine rejection of the love that act is supposed to represent. The eventual result is Pain Behavior, whether physical pain is involved or not.

Another result is guaranteed as well: lowered self-esteem. From the moment we feel unwanted or inadequate, or find ourselves in fear of loss, we spiral downward into destructive stress with all its attendant anxiety and muscular tension.

Intimate Relationships and Self-Esteem

As you recover, it's vital that you explore any effects of past suffering on your most intimate relationship. Physical closeness is likely to have been lost. With that loss of intimacy, self-esteem often decreases, and with lowered self-esteem comes lowered self-confidence.

You're not alone in this negative cycle. Your lover has been just as deeply affected by your pain and Pain Behavior. He or she also has another consideration: What if you don't recover to the point where you can make love again? We're all looking for the validation that making love can bring; we all long to be accepted physically by the one we love. Without that validation, self-esteem slips another notch; self-denial sets our minds looking for rationales and justifications, few of which are positive.

A love partner is very likely to see your inability to respond sexually as a personal rejection. We feel we're being denied sex because the other person no longer loves us, because we're no longer desirable. Wounded by this rejection, the physically well lover can go right into Pain Behavior: withdrawal, avoidance, escape. Both parties are being punished, and both are punishing. This is the process that results in the masochistic attitudes involved in Pain Behavior. Both parties have reached "victim" status. Feeling like victims, they act like victims. "You don't love me anymore" becomes the subtext of most conversations.

As long as we look upon sex as proof of love, we're missing the whole point. If we think of it as something apart from the whole relationship, intimacy is impossible. Bodies become objects to be used; orgasm ends interest. All of which is a waste of time, energy and love. But there is a positive alternative—one that only ignorance denies.

Building Intimacy

Even a sufferer on Level One can begin to build intimacy back into a love relationship. This is as true of physical contact as of emotional contact. Physical ability may be limited, but the degree of intention isn't. Making love is not just having sex; it's a whole-person, whole-relationship process.

Male or female, we all inhabit bodies structured to experience every sensual perception to the point of ecstasy. Even if our erogenous awareness has been dulled by pain, there are other senses that stimulate desire. Sound, sight, taste and smell help to set the stage for resensitizing our bodies. Touching, stroking or massaging can all reveal erogenous areas we never knew existed. The more we involve the senses, the more profound any experience becomes.

Sexual intimacy, however, is just one part of the picture. How you act toward your lover throughout the day is the only foreplay that makes a lasting difference. Even an expert at stimulating physical intimacy can be the most undesirable person alive if his or her aim is dominance or subversion in the relationship. If you're playing an "I win/you lose" game, you've already lost.

The Problem of "Performance"

For most men and women, the biggest stumbling block in creating intimacy on the physical level is "performance." Instead of keeping centered on what's happening at the moment (and responding naturally to that experience), "performers" act out what they think is expected of them. This disconnects them from the moment, makes them role players instead of lovers. Spontaneity and trust are more meaningful in love than passion and performance.

The Problem of Communication

Good communication in every shared area of life is the single ground rule for creating intimacy on the mental/emotional level. If such communication doesn't characterize the relationship, it's in trouble. Being willing to honestly discuss making love opens the door to discussing any other subjects that have been denied full disclosure. Such willingness means that each partner has truly accepted the other as a trusted equal.

As a couple, progress toward unconditional acceptance of body, mind and spirit means that the life you share will be enhanced beyond your dreams. And as with all accomplishment, success is a result—not a goal.

I think of the word "spirit" as pertaining to our power of choice. Choice takes place within the brain, of course, but that doesn't make it anatomical. The brain is the environment of the mind just as the body is the environment of the brain. If there is any human process which clearly indicates individual integrity, it is our power to choose a new behavior rather than to simply react according to past patterns. We don't have to accept defeat; we can always will to win. If this weren't the case, no one would get better.

The process of success is clear. To achieve any goal, we need education, motivation and the physical ability to achieve what we desire. It all begins with education. Should you be unfamiliar with the work of Masters and Johnson, do yourself a favor and read their work. Pioneers in the clinical aspect of sexual dysfunction, their *The Pleasure Bond—A New Look at Sexuality and Commitment* has helped many couples learn to function normally. Even couples who believe they *are* functioning normally would benefit from exploring further ways of enhancing their intimacy in making love.

In addition, there are many recent books, such as Alex Comfort's *The Joy of Sex,* which takes sex out of the closet in a positive and poetic way. These books emphasize sensitizing the act of love. Do all you can to discover more about your own body and that of your partner. Coming to grips with sexuality is coming to grips with an important part of yourself.

The Positions That Are Best for You

On Level One, a loving touch in any form is always safe *if* you've done your preparation mentally and physically. Even a bedridden person can return a loving touch.

Partially Ambulatory people (Level Two) can, with appropriate preparation, add oral love to loving touch. Depending on where they are on the road to recovery, actual penetration is possible—but that requires certain adaptations. The traditional "missionary position" puts terrific pressure on a woman's pelvis and lower spine. Do not employ this position in your condition, even if it's the one you're used to. The last thing either partner needs right now is a painful experience that might cause one or the other to quit before success is attained.

The "spoons position" is best and safest for Level Two people. In this position, the lovers lie on their sides, knees drawn up toward the stomach, bodies molded together, somewhat like two spoons fitting one inside the other. In this way, both backs will be supported and carry very little weight. Most movement will be flexion, which usually does not aggravate pain. Either partner can stop movement at any time without having to bear the other's weight. This is a gentle, loving position, not conducive to violent or vigorous movement. What's more, after sex you can go to sleep without changing position. That's important, because, like loving touch, holding is healing.

Other positions are available, depending on your willingness to experiment. Discover alternative positions and use them. Our only limits are the ones we impose upon ourselves. Success breeds success, whether it's in lovemaking, attitude reconstruction, weight loss or the ability to return to a job or profession. To most of us, reestablishing a loving relationship provides motivation for progress in every other area of life.

Again, at this stage in the recovery process, orgasm is a luxury, not a goal. The goal is rediscovering your sensuality. If at any time pain warns you to stop—*stop!* And should that happen before orgasm, show the same loving gratitude as if you'd climaxed. Lie close, touch, enjoy each other's presence and talk about the next time. If you've communicated your needs in advance, stopping before climax will present no problem.

Visualization:
Create What You Want in Making Love

Once you've decided what you can do, you'll need to set some realistic goals and do some necessary preparation. Visualization is your beginning point. Candace's story spells out in detail her use of visualization to preprogram success into each step of recovery in making love. With your goal in mind, put yourself into a relaxed state and visualize the actions required from beginning, to middle, to end. Approach it as a controlled activity, preprogramming any needed relaxation technique as a reinforcement.

Focus on sensations as you visualize; imagine in vivid detail all the sounds, sights, smells and touching involved. Become fascinated with as many sense images as come to mind. Imagine your body's response to your lover's touch. Set your mind free to become more and more aware of all sensation.

Should thoughts of past pain come to mind, disconnect them. Keep your full attention on savoring the sweetness of all that love can be. Allow yourself to be loved; allow yourself to love. Experience it fully. Repeat the process of preprogramming through visualization until it feels natural. Then is the time to turn your imaginings into action.

On the physical level, stretch-test all movements involved in achieving your goal, then set exercise goals and quotas as appropriate. Follow through so that your body matches your mind in terms of preparation.

Make the Right to Love a Rite of Love

Making love should be as special as the love that prompts it. Anticipation is enhanced by other preparations than those just described. There are the esthetics of the setting to be considered. Create the best environment for loving—music, your favorite scent, the lighting of the room, its temperature. Your visualization will tell you how to do this.

But beyond such considerations, keep in mind that the intimacy you're aiming for depends upon your attitude throughout the days preceding love. The more you show your partner an accepting, caring response, the more that person will want to share lovemaking with you.

After orgasm, relax and take time to allow that relaxing energy to radiate throughout your body, your entire being. While you're letting that wonderful sense of deep, peaceful relaxation release the tensions of life's pain, be aware that this relaxation is healing more than your body. It's helping heal the pain your suffering has inflicted on your partner, too.

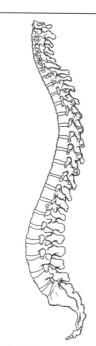

Reaching Out: How to Build Your Own Recovery Group

Recovery from prolonged pain is not unlike recovery from alcoholism. Like alcoholics, backaholics have numerous motivational problems. Dependence on medication substitutes for alcohol in chronic back suffering, and over the years the effect on the system is just as addictive. Like alcoholics, most backaholics don't realize they're succumbing to a degenerative process of body, mind and spirit. Believing that pain is their only problem, they justify making no effort to get better.

This is why the buddy system proves invaluable. Enthusiastic encouragement, whether from friends or family, helps personal motivation. Better yet, if someone exercises along with you, there's an added incentive to meet exercise quotas and attain exercise goals. It gives you someone with whom to share your feelings, your fears and your progress.

That's one of the reasons we created Postural Therapeutics, the first outpatient back rehabilitation clinic in the country. At the heart of our program was the realization that back sufferers needed an organized support group—people who shared the same affliction and desire to get better.

The clinic also offers group sessions in each of the three recovery basics: education, motivation and physical exercise to increase Level of Activity. I'd like to share in detail the components of the program we created so you can apply them to your own recovery regimen. Especially if you're on your own during this difficult time, you can use this information to enhance and hasten getting better. It all begins with finding out as much as you can about your condition.

Education

At Postural Therapeutics, we include half an hour of education with every one and a half-hour session. During this 30 minutes, we share physical skills training (such as correct methods to lift, bend, etc.) as well as information about the spine's structure—how it works and what goes wrong. There's a good deal of information on back muscles, too, along with other muscle groups that work in concert with back muscles in activities like walking and reaching. The effects of various medications are studied; so is the absolute importance of weaning away from them. We also deal with the psychological aspects of pain management.

Some education sessions are group raps with open discussions about pain and Pain Behavior. There's also biofeedback training and other relaxation skills for handling pain and developing dominion over fear of pain.

Motivation

Motivation is the key to getting better. Our program is designed to provide an upbeat atmosphere patients are glad to enter, a pleasant place staffed with pleasant, positive people whose sole purpose is to promote recovery. That's a real boost to a patient's personal motivation.

An even greater boost is being part of a group of others determined to recover. It's no coincidence that our groups are coeducational. Men and women quickly decide to improve visually in each others' company. Tummies are tucked in, makeup is applied, everyone becomes more weight-conscious and tries to look his or her best.

We also make no distinction between different Levels of Activity when it comes to group exercise. All levels work together. Such groups recognize and appreciate attitudinal progress as much as physical progress. There's an aura of increasing self-assurance. "How I can" becomes the subject of conversation, improvement being the basic subtext.

Exercise

At our clinic, groups do half an hour of mat exercise and another half hour in the pool, with people on Level Two exercising right alongside Level Three and Four people. A competitive spirit starts to manifest itself. Yet everyone understands and appreciates exactly what everyone else has been through and what they're experiencing now. Also, one's peers are far more candid and direct than many therapists when it comes to prodding progress out of overly cautious or despairing members of the group. Such prodding is given with empathy and received with respect. It's hard not to get better when you're surrounded by such good examples.

Following a physical exercise regimen on your own is entirely up to you. Even if you can overcome the initial discomfort and fear of pain, you still have to deal with the lonely boredom of endless repetitions. Without the buddy system to provide support, encouragement and honest prodding, it's easy to slack off, procrastinate, even skip exercise altogether.

That's why I suggest that you sign up with a local rehabilitation clinic. As of this writing, there are more than 5,000 outpatient back clinics in the United States. Almost every major hospital and university has one. None are cost-free, but many such programs are covered by medical compensation. As a matter of fact, in the majority of clinics, you'll need a physician's recommendation or prescription to enroll. That should be no problem, though, because conservative therapy, aggressively applied, is becoming doctors' treatment of choice for most back problems today.

Not all rehabilitation facilities have access to a pool for water exercise, but that's not vital; increasing your mat exercise time from 30 minutes to an hour will serve essentially the same purpose. The only thing you'll be missing will be the relaxing warmth of exercising in a heated pool. And even that isn't denied you if you can make arrangements with a local spa or pool for water exercise in addition to your mat regimen at the rehab clinic. All exercise speeds progress; the more you do, the sooner you'll see results.

The Buddy System at Home

If there are no outpatient rehab facilities nearby, you're still not out of luck if you're married or involved in a relationship. Even if your partner isn't suffering from a back problem, the exercise will be therapeutic. What's more, you'll be sharing an experience that can enrich the relationship.

Family members and/or friends can substitute if you have no such loving relationship at this time; but in one form or another, you need a positive support group to maintain your motivation. Those who recover totally on their own from serious back conditions (especially after long-term chronic suffering) are a distinct minority. But if you *are* a person alone, without a loved one, family or friends who can devote some time to sharing in your recovery program, you still have another option. This alternative is not only viable and positive, it's also one of the best ways to take responsibility for your recovery.

Form Your Own Recovery Group

With nearly one out of three people in America suffering from a bad back, you're bound to be acquainted with a number of fellow sufferers among your friends, associates or co-workers. Let them know you're forming a recovery group. Explain that it will feature education about the back, discussions on maintaining motivation and a regular program of exercise to increase Levels of Activity.

You might post a notice on bulletin boards in your neighborhood or where you work. You might even put a small ad in your local newspaper. The ideal size for a recovery group is from eight to ten people, so it shouldn't be difficult to find people who want to join you in getting better.

What You Need in Terms of Equipment

No special equipment is required—only the space needed for exercising. Should you have access to a heated pool, so much the better, but that's not a major requirement. The most important factor for success is group involvement.

The 30-minute education portion of your 90-minute meeting will require your group to locate appropriate informational materials. You might want to reach out beyond books and magazine articles to include videotapes or films on the back's anatomy, function and recovery. Again, your local library is a good source for such materials, and so is your physician.

If you have some difficulty securing a biofeedback device or learning how to use it, remember that even without the actual equipment, working with your self-created mental biofeedback mechanism can produce the desired results.

When it comes to relaxation training, your group members are an excellent resource. Each one can take a turn, for example, at bringing in a new book or cassette tape on relaxation skills. Likewise, each might be responsible for a presentation on the back's anatomy and treatment.

The more each group member accepts responsibility for helping create the program, the more successful each member will be in getting better. Becoming your own authorities and instructors is a superb way of increasing assurance, independence and self-esteem.

The Best Environment

All you really need in order to get started is a pleasant space, big enough for exercising. Attitude is much more important than decor, but environment often sets the tone. The more pleasant and attractive the space, the more pleasant and attractive it will be to attend group recovery sessions. Here again, everyone can pitch in.

Have beautiful things around to look at—paintings, flowers, travel posters, etc. If at all possible, have a large mirror or mirror panels in the room. It really helps when you can see yourselves in action, when you can see (rather that just *feel*) your physical abilities increasing. Exercise becomes a reward in itself. You get the itch to look better in general, and this is a real Revolving Reward, especially for overweight people.

You might like to add color to your sessions by suggesting that group members purchase exercise clothing in their favorite hues. The available stock in such clothing is a rainbow of colors these days; in fact, drab gray or navy sweatsuits seem to be as passé as wrist corsages and rumble seats. Don't overlook the importance of music when planning your group environment. Exercising to music makes exertion easier, since the music itself has a clear beginning, middle and end. Your music is limited only by two considerations: mood and imagination. The mood should be positive, upbeat. It's a good idea to have each member furnish tapes or records for the exercise part of your program. In doing so, everyone comes to know one another on a more personal basis. It's another step toward involvement—and another Revolving Reward.

Bring Along the Right Attitude

If you've taken the initiative in organizing the group, they'll be looking for you to set the tone. Go for equality—equal participation, equal responsibility and equal authority from all hands. Remember, chronic sufferers have usually relinquished authority and feel they must depend on someone other than themselves for mobility, motivation and medication. Since one of the major purposes of your recovery group is to reestablish each person as his or her own authority for getting better, your group needs continued appreciation for progress (not sympathy for backsliding) as well as encouragement when the going gets tough.

As long as each member is treated as an equal (and treats others the same way), as long as there is respect, honest encouragement and appreciation, your group will grow in Well Behavior. After all, there are no excuses a backaholic can come up with that other recovering backaholics haven't used themselves. As peers, they've shared the same pain and the same problems.

In such an atmosphere of appreciation, encouragement and equality, people feel better and they get better. After a few sessions—meeting two times a week—you'll probably find you're not only working with other back sufferers, you're working with *friends*. Many of them will share that feeling and many will be feeling—perhaps for the first time in months, possibly years—that they're back in the social swim with people who genuinely care about them.

Get in Tune for Toning

Your group will be made up of both sexes at varying Levels of Activity, but all levels should do the *same* exercises—each to the best of his or her own ability and according to individual goals and quotas.

It's valuable for the entire group to establish those goals and quotas during your first meeting. It's also valuable to write these goals and quotas down in order to know when they've been attained. Since such a record is best kept in one place, you might choose to create a group recovery journal, just as you may have created a personal journal.

With all the above in mind, there's one more area I'd like to touch on before we leave the subject of what you plan *in general* for your recovery group. This is a very special area of concern, one that affects group environment, attitude and exercise. Most of all, it's the key to a positive group dynamic and the best boost of motivation you can have.

The Healing Power of Laughter

Laughter is something we pretty much take for granted—except when we're flat on our backs, suffering with chronic pain. At such times, life is hardly amusing, and laughter is mostly a memory. American poet Ella

Wheeler Wilcox put it this way: "Laugh and the world laughs with you, cry and you cry alone." The latter portion of that statement, unfortunately, is not true, for when one family member suffers chronic pain, a cloak of sorrow falls over the entire household.

Fortunately, Mrs. Wilcox hit the nail on the head with her first seven words. Laughter almost inevitably breeds laughter. And as a form of positive muscular exertion, it doubles as a physical exercise and mental relaxation. Beyond all else, laughter is the perfect accompaniment to getting better.

In his best-selling book, *Anatomy of an Illness,* author Norman Cousins documents his own battle with a crippling disease of the spine, a disease which, several specialists assured him, would lead to his death within 18 months. Due to a collagen-related illness, the connective tissue of his spine was deteriorating. Collagen, remember, forms the basic component of spinal discs that cushions vertebrae from coming in contact with one another. Mr. Cousins refused to accept his death sentence and began investigating alternatives to the bedridden existence foisted upon him by this degenerative disease. Working with his personal physician, he explored many different approaches to possible recovery. The one that worked best, amazingly enough, was laughter.

In order to reinforce his sometimes wavering positive attitude while he was in the hospital, Cousins's friend, Alan Funt, sent film clips of some of the funniest segments from his long-running TV comedy show, "Candid Camera." Even though Cousins was depressed, bedridden, unable to sleep, wracked with pain and heavily medicated, he found he could still laugh. In fact, ten minutes of belly laughter had such a relaxing, anaesthetic effect, he went to sleep and slept for two pain-free hours. When he woke, he had a plan. His private nurse was taught to operate the film projector and the Marx Brothers joined "Candid Camera" as staples in his innovative self-treatment regimen. So did humorous writings by favorite comedic authors. In addition to the films, his nurse read aloud from the *Subtreasure of American Humor* and Max Eastman's *The Enjoyment of Laughter.* Cousins found that a few minutes of laughter relaxed his mind and body and eased his pain.

Within a week, he had weaned himself off all medication including sleeping pills. In eight weeks' time, this man who had been given a death verdict was back at work. Not that it was easy; there was pain and severe physical limitation. It took months before he was able to reach higher than his shoulders, years before he had full range of motion in his neck.

"Laughter therapy" wasn't his only mode of treatment, but Norman Cousins chooses to believe that laughter helped his recovery—and so do I.

On the physical level, laughter compels us to fully expel all air from our lungs, then gulp in all the air those lungs can hold. In effect, it produces the same benefit as controlled breathing, which permits us to gain a maximum supply of oxygen. Relaxation results from both activities.

Another positive physical feature of laughter is that it gives the organs in the thorax a real workout, not to mention the abdominal muscles themselves. Body-involving laughter serves much the same purpose as do half sit-ups when it comes to exercise. And it has the advantage of being totally enjoyable, involuntary exercise. In fact, the uncontrollable nature of laughter is its best feature; we extend our physical limits without even thinking about it.

On the mental level, laughter relieves tension in exactly the same way. What we see or hear that provokes laughter takes us totally outside our usual focus. For the length of time we're laughing, anxiety and pain fade from consciousness. Even after laughter stops, we tend to go on chuckling from the memory of what amused us. Our mood is lighter, our outlook more positive.

That's why I suggest that you make your sessions brighter by preprogramming for laughter. Play a cassette or record of your favorite comedian before the session starts. Or show the videotape of a film that guarantees guffaws. At Postural Therapeutics, we've found that Laurel and Hardy are ideal companions with whom to get better. Not only are their antics funny to most people, they're even educational. No one does things the *wrong* way, physically speaking, as well as Laurel and Hardy. We show their film "The Music Box" regularly as an example of how *not* to lift, bend, reach, stand, walk, fall, stretch—practically anything that has to do with motions affecting the back.

Invite group members to take turns bringing in laughter-provoking material for each session. And encourage everyone to start watching genuinely amusing television programs and going to really funny films. The more we laugh, the easier it is to laugh at our own foibles, inadequacies and pain. Laughter is truly a gift in healing.

Ground Rules for the Group Dynamic

During your initial organizational meeting, I feel it's a good idea to achieve agreement on some basic ground rules. Once accepted, they make for a smooth-flowing, positive group dynamic. Each is important in that it focuses the individual on personal responsibility for getting better.

Take Responsibility for Your Own Recovery

Each member must take full responsibility for his or her individual progress, as well as for handling any pain involved in physical exercise along the way. (Part of that responsibility, of course, is clearing in advance with a physican that it's all right to participate in a recovery group.)

Promote Well Behavior

Pain Behavior is to be acknowledged and dealt with whenever it crops up, but the focus of the group is on getting better. Pain is a given, so the subject of pain is meaningless except when a member can announce a positive improvement or when new ways to manage pain are being introduced as part of your educational sessions.

Celebrate Each Step of Progress

Encouragement and appreciation should be given for any improvement, both individually and by the entire group. On the other side of the coin, backsliding will be acknowledged in the same direct, honest and empathetic way. Among peers who have chosen to recover, honest praise and honest criticism go hand in hand. Each person's success is the group's success, and the group's success depends on each of its members being successful.

Recognize That Everyone Is Equal

Each group member is equally important, gets equal time to share feelings and concerns, and is equally responsible for seeing to it that same right is extended to all other members. No one is the "authority" for the group; all participate equally in the responsibilities of research, education, reportage and physical exercise. The goal is getting better, individually and as a group.

Once you've agreed on the ground rules, you're ready to go into action. At your first meeting, you'll find it valuable to give each group member the opportunity—for the first and last time—to review his or her individual case history. This will enable each member to define current Levels of Activity and to set recovery goals.

Then it's time to set immediate goals for physical exercise and specific quotas of exercise repetitions to attain those goals. Since the individual alone sets those goals and quotas there should be no discussion, only acceptance and an appropriate notation made in the group recovery journal. Also, while goals for physical recovery are important, setting goals to get better mentally are just as vital.

Acknowledging Pain Behavior is crucial in your group dynamic. Backaholics need encouragement and positive support to keep the mental turnaround alive in mind and heart. While the group doesn't need specifics verbalized, each member might well consider improving a close relationship at home or on the job as part of the recovery process. Whatever relationship has been most affected by Pain Behavior is the logical place to begin. Such mental turnaround goals should be briefly identified and logged in the journal.

After the organizational meeting, twice-weekly sessions should be the rule. Again, I suggest you follow the general format we've developed at Postural Therapeutics:

- Half an hour of education on back basics, relaxation skills, etc.

- Half an hour of mat exercise and half an hour of water exercise. If no pool is available, do an hour's worth of mat exercising. Just take a relaxation break after the first 30 minutes.

In addition, your group may find it profitable to follow up formal sessions with another half hour of practicing relaxation skills.

If your group is running effectively, your members will be glad to attend sessions and eager to see each other again. They'll be grateful for their own progress and the progress of their peers. Opening on an upbeat note relaxes the tensions that may have built up between sessions. Closing with laughter extends the group's positive mood into the future. After all, you're discovering that there *is* life after (and during) pain. As far as I'm concerned, you're doing something truly heroic, truly life-affirming. And you're setting a winning example for any other back sufferers with whom your group might come in contact.

Self and Group Evaluation

Another feature of the program is a review of progress toward goals set during the first session. Once more, remember that the individual is the only authority when it comes to setting and attaining any goal, but group feedback is very important. With people working on recovery together, there's a lot of therapeutic value in group evaluation.

In a group that encourages positive results and discourages negative feedback, patients become their own therapists to a very significant degree. At Postural Therapeutics, we have professional counselors on staff, but we find that our patients monitor themselves and other recoverers as a matter of course. No one understands better the problems involved than those who've been through them. Peer pressure and approval is one of life's most powerful incentives.

Hold an evaluation session once a month. Acknowledge progress, help with any problems that might have surfaced and reset goals and quotas as appropriate. These new goals, quotas and mental turnaround targets should be duly noted in the group's journal.

Togetherness as Therapy

Since any activity is physical exercise, an active social life promotes a speedier recovery. Why not initiate a plan whereby your group includes some social activity on a regular basis? You could take turns hosting dinners in your homes, for example. Preparing a meal has added advantages from the physical exercise point of view. Shopping for a meal, putting it together and serving it is valuable exertion. So is cleaning up afterward. Of course, there's nothing wrong with asking for help from other members of the group. Most people are more than willing to pitch in.

Then there are plays and films to see, new restaurants to investigate. Pick places and entertainments you can dress up for. That's an added incentive and imparts more glamour to any activity. Whatever you choose to do socially, do as much as possible together. The isolation, loneliness and depression that accompanies chronic back pain is the same for everyone in the group. It's healing to realize none of you is alone anymore.

There are many reasons to include your family in a recovery group social activity. They make a great addition because their pride in your improvement will boost everybody's spirits. You might include them in some of your educational sessions as well. It's good for them to understand the whys and wherefores of the overall program. After suffering along with your Pain Behavior, they probably need some recovery skills as much as you do.

In outpatient rehab clinics around the country, this is becoming the rule. The husband or wife of the sufferer is requested to share appropriate parts of the program. This extends in some instances beyond the educational sessions to include actual exercise itself. Your group may want to plan such inclusion shortly after you've settled into your formal format.

Another extension of activity might be to create a series of special sessions to discuss weight-control motivation, on-the-job exercises or any subject pertinent to recovery. Take turns chairing these meetings; being in charge of part of the program is a plus for self-esteem and self-confidence.

Reach Out to Other Sufferers

If you've been helped, help others. There must be people in your area who've been bedridden for months. Completely removed from life's mainstream, most of them are suffering limitations which you know can cripple more than their bodies. What would it be like if your group took on a project of outreach to such sufferers? Once you're sure of your own improvement, arrange to visit such a person. What you share might inspire that sufferer with renewed interest in getting better.

An outreach of this kind provides a twofold benefit for the recovery group. First, it reminds them what getting *worse* holds in store, hence it doubles incentive to improve on their own behalf. Second, it will bring your group closer together as a unit dedicated to setting the example that recovery, to whatever degree, is possible.

In your collective recovery, there's hope for everyone. More than offering hope, however, you'll be setting a pattern of self-directed outpatient health improvement that might benefit hundreds in your community.

Regular Medical Checkups: Proof of Improvement

Regular medical checkups are a must in your recovery. Not only will they underscore your success, they'll give you the opportunity to stay abreast of current medical information and new techniques for physical exercise.

The Voice of Authority

Once the group sessions are rolling, you may want to invite some health authorities to address your group on special subjects. Conservative therapy, aggressively applied, is making giant strides in the field of returning back sufferers to full activity.

The same is true with innovative approaches to exercise. To be aware of these advances, you may find it valuable to invite a physical therapist to explain such exercises. Perhaps you could interest a biofeedback technician in what you're doing and experience an actual clinical process of biofeedback. A local psychologist might address your group regarding a deeper understanding of Pain Behavior.

There are informed people in every area of your concern who can be sources of needed information. Like all activity, every outreach gives you more assurance, confidence and self-esteem.

How Long Should Your Group Continue?

At Postural Therapeutics, we've found that depending on the Level of Activity of those involved, 2 weekly visits for a period of two months produces significant progress. We've had members return to work after an average number of 16 visits. Many chronic sufferers want to continue beyond any set time span for the added motivation that camaraderie can give them.

Let your group set its own beginning, middle and end. And even when the group does dissolve, it's hard to imagine that you'll be out of touch. What you've shared has been more than education, motivation and exercise. You've shared one of the most significant experiences life offers: You've *grown* together. You've cared about each other. You've talked progress and you've seen it happen. Most of all, you have friends who are partners, equals in effort and accomplishment. That's an experience to be treasured.

In fact, that experience is so vital you may want to repeat it, working with a new group. All you've learned, all you've profited from in your first group will be even more effective with a second, possibly a third and fourth.

Working with another group of recoverers gives you a regular health and muscle maintenance program. It's also the best insurance that you'll never go through such immobility and pain again. It serves as a constant reminder that taking responsibility for the care and maintenance of your back is a lifetime occupation.

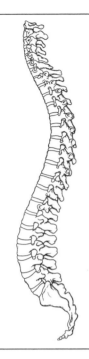

Creating a Relaxing Lifestyle

CHAPTER 12

Most back problems result from destructive stress, and most stress results from mishandled emotions and relationships. Thus, our best health insurance is to create a relaxing lifestyle. Such a lifestyle is both the solution and prevention for any physical pain you may now be suffering or may suffer in the future.

I'm not talking about anything as simple as two-week vacations, a couple of martinis before dinner or going to bed early to get your beauty sleep. I'm suggesting that a relaxing lifestyle exists on two levels—the physical and the mental. Of the two, what we think and feel is more important, since the body is the reflection of our state of mind, our attitudes, our knowledge and our ignorance.

Mentally, a relaxing lifestyle is achieved through Well Behavior. It's reinforced by introspection and honesty about the problems that produce the pain of life. Sessions of sand dune therapy are needed regularly to identify and defuse the stressors we allow to overwhelm our wellbeing. Physically, the regular use of programmed relaxation can help release the muscle tension that results from mental stress. And, in the long run, regular physical exercise (preceded and followed by relaxation) dispels that tension through the cycle of constructive stress.

This is a full-time job for all of us. To the degree that we succeed, we stay well. Our bodies stay younger and our minds remain clear to turn stumbling blocks into stepping-stones. But such behavior flies in the face of all the problems our previous ignorance has set in our path. As we were growing up, few of us were lucky enough to become educated on how to deal with life's problems or relationships. But we learned many negative reaction patterns, in much the same way as we acquire Pain Behavior. Our way of handling tough situations or emotions becomes habitual. Changing those patterns isn't easy. It takes conscious control, exercised at least as often as we exercise our bodies, to achieve and maintain mental mastery over the stressors in our lives.

It is in our relationships that the greatest stressors manifest themselves. When communication is strained, when we fear failure or loss in a relationship or on the job, stressors loom overwhelming. Which is why *now* is the time to begin bridging those communication gaps. More important, it's time to conduct all of our relationships with the skills that insure that those gaps won't occur in the future—or at least that we're not responsible for the miscommunication that does occur.

Coping Through Communication

Coping skills are only now being researched and developed, so don't flog yourself for ignorance in this department. Instead, take responsibility for finding out what they are and how to use them. You don't lack opportunity. There are excellent seminars available to the public and excellent classes in communication skills being offered in colleges and universities across the country.

In addition, almost every major communication skills program has its own published text, with the step-by-step how-tos clearly explained in black and white. When you find a book that makes sense to you, learn more about the author and the programs he or she has created.

One of the pioneers in this field is Thomas Gordon, M.D., whose Parent Effectiveness Training was the first in a series of valuable books on communication-coping skills. Dr. Gordon's subsequent work applies those skills to leadership and teaching. His popularization of psychological concepts developed by Carl Rogers, among others, has been the basis for increased quality in communication for millions. I mention Dr. Gordon as a starting point only. There are scores of valuable works on the subject.

Through study, observation and some sand dune soul searching, I've found there is one ground rule to good communication: honest acceptance of responsibility for how I say what I say—especially in stressful situations. Granted, it isn't easy to practice 100 percent of the time. But to the degree I manage to employ this rule, I find it's a lot easier to maintain good communication.

Translate "You-Messages" into "I-Language"

In stressful situations, accepting full responsibility for how I say what I say means using a different kind of language. Our usual response to problems or pressures is to fix blame or shame upon the apparent antagonist. This most often takes the form of You-Messages such as: It is your fault, you're wrong, you don't understand, you've hurt my feelings, you've failed to meet my expectations, etc. Such attacks make a person feel defensive, and an already deteriorating situation becomes worse. You-Messages are the language of Pain Behavior.

The mental turnaround principle applies to the communication process as well as to recovery. As long as we believe that pain is the only problem, we have no control over getting better. In communication problems, as long as we believe that another person is the cause of what we feel, there's no way to seek solutions. At the heart of getting better is the decision to choose a different response than how we've responded in the past.

To improve personal communication, I-Language is the way to go. I-Language is a consciously chosen style of response that tells only what *I* feel and what *my* goals are. There's no blame or shame, just authentic feeling and a clear direction. Let me give you an example:

You-Message Statement: "You make me furious with your constant complaining and all your excuses. Why can't you shape up and act like a human being for a change? You're destroying this relationship!"

I-Language Translation: "I'm really upset about what's going on; in fact, I'm downright angry. What I want is to get a clear picture of what I can do to improve this relationship. It means a lot to me or I wouldn't feel so bad. I want to make it work."

Obviously there's a real contrast in the effect I-Language has on people. I-Language acknowledges your authentic feeling and states the goal without getting into anyone's emotions other than your own. It clearly states your intention and bypasses judgment or blame or shame.

By eliminating the chain reaction triggered by the word "you," the negative part of the situation is partially defused and chances are that a positive communication can take place. Drop You-Messages from stressful situations. Take responsibility for thinking, not just reacting. Make the mental turnaround; you'll find it works.

And it works because the very act of choosing to choose a different way of expressing yourself means you're using the front brain rather than the rear brain reactor bank. Making the conscious choice to rethink You-Messages and translate them into responsible, authentic I-Language leaves you more cool and collected. It also cuts down all the time wasted by excusing and justifying.

Consciously and unconsciously, you've already started to use I-Language if you've joined a recovery group. The process of that group's dynamic depends on honesty with self, goal setting and goal getting as well as exercise and improved relationships. I-Language encourages the positive, discourages the negative and keeps your focus on getting better.

Find a Relaxing Environment

No matter where or how you live, you can live with greater relaxation if you upgrade that environment so that you're surrounded by the colors, sounds and things that make you feel at peace and at one with yourself. This statement is no generality; it's as specific as your individual taste.

I'm frequently amazed at how little care some people take to surround themselves with an environment they really want to be part of. And yet creating that kind of environment is as important as taking care of your physical appearance. Just as your body is the environment in which your brain operates and reflects your basic mental attitudes, your place of living indicates those attitudes in exactly the same way. Are you surrounded by disarray and disorder? If you are, how can you be pleased to be there? Does the decor reflect what you feel is beautiful? If not, it can't relax you. Do you spend hours in front of the television set, watching and listening to other people's ideas and opinions? If so, you're denying yourself the exploration of your own.

In recovery, you've reestablished a positive connection between mind and body. Let that reflect in your outer environment. Complete the connection. Make your place of living worth living in. Use your own ideas about color and design. Upgrading your environment can be as significant as increasing your Level of Activity through exercise. And the activity involves just as much effort as any other physical exercise—another Revolving Reward.

Another way to develop a relaxing environment is through music. Music is essential for setting a mood, and can even promote a meditative state of mind. Psychological research has demonstrated that certain forms of music are not only more relaxing than others, they can also foster easy learning. A whole new approach to rapid comprehension called "Super Learning" is based on this notion and uses specific kinds of music in the background while basic information is presented.

Composers from the Baroque period—Bach, Haydn, Handel, Vivaldi and Albinoni—are excellent for this practice. The beginning-middle-end style of their work meets the requirements of both mental and physical exercise. Also, their theme-and-variation approach expands mental process into imagination, releasing images that draw the mind away from stress.

If you haven't developed a taste for such cerebral compositions, you might investigate the works of more romantic composers, beginning with Mozart and Beethoven, then moving into Brahms or Rachmaninoff. The concertos of these artists are particularly useful to a meditative and relaxed state of mind.

There's also a modern movement toward music *specifically* designed to relax mind and body. Halpern and Larkin are excellent examples; their compositions are as spontaneous and quietly colorful as they are haunting. Taking much from the raga-forms of India, some of the Beatles' music and a good deal of Paul Horn's, they express the meditative state in melodic variation. Investigate, experiment, expand your usual musical taste to include classic composers and the new wave of meditative music.

Develop Your Creativity

All of the previous categories offer you new creative options, but I'm speaking here of developing new interests, new hobbies—especially ones in which you work with your hands. In effect, I'm suggesting that you create your own occupational therapy program. But it goes beyond that.

During recovery, working with your hands gives you a whole new spectrum of sensation to experience. Working with wood, clay, macramé, soapstone, silver or bread dough is truly therapeutic. Touching unfamiliar textures becomes a form of fascination that takes your mind off pain and provides a concentrated focus on the moment. People who bake their own bread testify to the healing feelings related to that activity, just as working at a lathe provides the same calm focus to others.

Beyond therapy, developing a new hobby gives you the opportunity to create something only you can do—something for which you are the only authority. Many people discover a love of watercolor or oil painting during recovery. Working with color, creating form and feeling through such media can become a vocational way of life. So can sculpting in clay, working with ceramics, sketching, or designing your own greeting cards. The list is endless, and so are the benefits.

Creative expression is the most absorbing of all mental activity. At the same time, it relaxes us from the usual cares and troubles of the day, energizing us in mind, body and spirit. All of us have this creative potential. Maybe yours will be found in learning to play a musical instrument so that you can create your own music for relaxation.

Every one of us has latent talents we've long ignored. What are yours? Reflect and discover. You may find yourself developing a new avocation, an activity that can change your outlook or maybe even your entire life. If it's taken a painful back episode to give you the chance to create the kind of life you really want, then your pain had a purpose. It made you think about *you*, the real you—your own creative self.

Develop Your Sense of Humor

You don't need Laurel and Hardy reruns to keep you in stitches. The funniest person I know looks back at me from the mirror every morning. In time, I hope you'll feel that way about yourself.

Not that people should chuckle or guffaw at us as we pass them on the street, but a true sense of humor is indeed the ability to laugh at our own foibles, frailties and faux pas. Laughing at another's clumsiness or ignorance is cruel, but laughing at our own failings is genuine acceptance of responsibility for what we do that's ridiculous. People who don't find themselves amusing live very dreary lives. Such an attitude of dour self-denial reflects in their "I win/you lose" approach to life. Yes, we all make mistakes, however perfect we want to be. Accepting those mistakes with laughter frees us to correct them. Denying such mistakes leads to self-justification and self-righteousness, both of which are triggers for destructive stress.

If you're experiencing an acute attack or a prolonged bout with chronic pain, you probably feel there isn't much to laugh at; amusement can seem petty when compared to the agony you suffer. On an emotional level, that's true, of course. Yet objectively—as Norman Cousins proved to his satisfaction—letting yourself laugh may be the turning point toward getting better. The very contrast to your current depressed state jars you out of Pain Behavior. Once you've let that happen, laughter may become addictive. Let it happen. It's the medication you need most right now—and always.

Relaxing the Body

I'd like to share some thoughts about creating a regimen of relaxation on the *physical* level. The kind of exercises I've outlined in this book is basic to recovery from back problems, but once you find you can take all those exercises in stride, you may choose to augment this program with alternative approaches to physical exercise.

Yoga

One of my patients once said, "After medication, meditation." While I don't necessarily endorse the philosophy involved in yoga, the mental and physical discipline involved is superb.

As controlled stretching exercise, yoga has no peer. Many people consider it the best form of exercise, and focus on it exclusively as their way of increasing their Level of Activity. And there are other positive aspects of yoga to be found in its meditative discipline and emphasis on controlled breathing.

Should you elect to experiment with yoga, go carefully. Don't undertake it alone or uninstructed. And let your instructor know what your Level of Activity is, what exercise you've been doing, and any physical limitations you experience.

Aerobic Dance, Running, Jogging and Walking

Unless you're at Level Four (Unrestricted Activity, Chronic Lower Back Pain), do *not* involve yourself with aerobic dance, running or jogging. In time—with your doctor's approval—you may look into them, but even then, be cautious. Aerobic dance puts your body through exertions that can cause flare-ups during recovery. It also puts a bounce into stretching motions that can endanger muscles.

Walking has far fewer variables than any other exercise. A *brisk* walk for half an hour does just as much for your body as jogging or running, without the attendant physical stress. It removes the *jarring* factor. As popular as jogging may be, it can produce as many problems as it solves. Take a brisk walk morning and evening; work one in at midday if you can. The more you walk, the more your muscles can rebalance and tone themselves naturally.

Reinvolvement with Sports

For those recoverers who long to resume a sporting life, the prognosis is positive. Most likely you'll have reached the upper echelons of Level Three or the lower rungs of Level Four before you'll receive your physician's approval. But even when you have medical permission, use caution.

If you didn't play racquetball before your back episode, you probably shouldn't attempt to do so now. On the other hand, if you've played tennis before, begin to play again. Of all intermediate sports, swimming is best during recovery. Perhaps your first move in the direction of return to sports might be extending your water exercises by swimming laps across the pool.

Always warm up with stretching exercises before tackling any sport. This is especially true if it's a team sport. Competitive sports stir emotion, and we find ourselves pushing beyond our limits. But blithely overstepping bounds is as dangerous to your back as overkill exertion. Be wise, play for enjoyment and approach the game as you would any controlled activity. Program relaxation before and after the game.

So pick a sport appropriate to your current Level of Activity, and reinvolve yourself only with a physician's approval. Once you're committed to a given sport, take the precaution of increasing your regular exercise regimen prior to actually playing. Do the additional on-the-job exercises recommended for weekend warriors as spelled out in Chapter 9. And don't skimp on equipment. Buy quality merchandise and take advantage of any technical improvements in sporting gear.

Continued Education, Motivation and Exercise

Maintaining the degree of recovery you've been able to attain depends on continued self-education, self-motivation and physical activity to increase your Level of Activity. These three recovery basics apply equally to preservation of your current status and to prevention of future back trouble. Don't think for a minute that exercise alone will forestall back flare-ups. A positive mental outlook—one that promotes positive handling of life's painful experiences—is every bit as important. And such an outlook depends upon an active, inquisitive, enthusiastic attitude based on Well Behavior.

The more you discover what's new (education), the more excited you'll feel (motivation) about getting involved with challenging new activities (exercise). The more you program relaxation into your life, the easier such new activities will be for you, mentally and physically. You'll *be* more, *do* more and *have* more as the result—which means that more new doors will open for expanding both interest and activity. What better example of the Revolving Reward System than the overall enhancement of your life?

Interest, Activity and Aging

As the years pass, following the pattern of continued education, motivation and physical exercise produces another benefit—longevity. While there's no surefire guarantee for this, your chances for staying alert and active as you age increase in direct ratio to your active participation in life itself.

People like Albert Schweitzer, Pablo Picasso, Eleanor Roosevelt, Georgia O'Keefe, Frank Lloyd Wright, George Washington Carver and choreographer Martha Graham are famous for having maintained active participation in their chosen fields well beyond their seventies. American primitive artist Grandma Moses was still painting at age 100. Cellist Pablo Casal performed well into his nineties.

What such people have in common is a vital interest in life and living. This élan was their primary motivating force. Naturally, without such powerful motivation, they could never have maintained the physical discipline that supported the energy level necessary to meet their goals.

Intense interest begins a cycle of constructive stress that leads to well-earned relaxation of both body and mind. Since aging itself is a degenerative condition, those who forestall it best are those who choose their challenges, work at optimum exertion and balance that activity with rest. When we turn destructive stress into constructive stress, we maintain a more youthful body, mind and spirit. Your recovery program sets the pattern for a longer, more happy and productive life.

Honor Your Mind and Body

Pain exists only to tell you that your body has a problem in need of attention. Paying attention to that pain for what it is—and nothing more—frees us to take the necessary corrective action.

It's much easier to identify physical than mental pain because physical symptoms can't be overlooked for very long. Mental pain masquerades in many guises, the most obvious of which is Pain Behavior.

To maintain and increase recovery, it's vital that we continue to acknowledge our Pain Behavior whenever it manifests itself. If we don't, its self-fulfilling prophecy is all too likely to transform into psycho-physiological pain and the whole pain-sustained-by-stress pattern begins again.

Honor what your body tells you with physical pain; also honor what you mind is telling you when you catch yourself acting out Pain Behavior. You need no recurrence of an acute attack or chronic condition. Use the early-warning signals of pain and/or Pain Behavior to recognize and defuse any such recurrence. By doing so, you're guaranteeing continued progress— and in the process you're honoring yourself.

Maintain Your Support System

On the most personal level of your life, apply your recovery insight to building your relationships in the same way you're building a new life. Be the kind of person you most admire—as a lover and as a friend. Let unconditional acceptance be your guideline. Let intimacy be your goal. Your home should be a place of healing for you and your loved ones, a place where you can relax together, grateful for the companionship you share. It can be that kind of place if you set the example of Well Behavior there.

Professionally as well, you need the best support system you can create. Maintaining Well Behavior on the job has many benefits, and building a more intimate relationship with people working around you pays off in positive attention and friendship. You'll find others more willing to cooperate, more willing to get motivated when you set the example of its benefits through your recovery.

I hope you'll have been part of a recovery group—either by way of a rehabilitation clinic or one of your own creation. Never lose touch with those who actively participated with you in the recovery process. They will remain your best examples, just as you are theirs, that recovery means having won an agonizing war—a war you need never fight again if you continue to do what's required to stay recovered.

Ever since we founded Postural Therapeutics, it's been my dream to inspire individuals to create their own recovery groups in locations where no other rehabilitation opportunity exists. I've even dreamed of forming a network of such groups all across the nation so that anywhere, anytime back sufferers needed a support group of recoverers from back problems, they'd have one near at hand. No one would have to suffer alone with all the confusion, self-doubt and agony that attend afflictions with no apparent clinical cause.

Organizing such a network could serve as a central information center for the latest data on recovery from back problems. More than that, it could become a prime motivational force to achieve recovery. As a paramedical extension of doctor-prescribed rehabilitation therapy, it could perform the same service to back sufferers as Alcoholics Anonymous has for alcoholics. After all, there are almost 80 million Americans who need the motivation and inspiration that are found only in a group that is singularly focused on recovery.

If I have the dream of forming such a network, chances are very good that others share the same vision. In time, this formation will happen, because human consciousness is changing. Instead of locking in on limitation, people everywhere are moving toward freedom in their lives and in their minds. Dreams have a way of coming true once they've been verbalized and shared. Certainly the need exists. There is no longer any excuse for suffering.

Victor Versus Victim

Morty Stein, to whom this book is dedicated, contracted polio as a child of eight. It left him a functional quadriplegic. But that wasn't all; Morty also had scoliosis—a crippling, twisting condition of the spine that would worsen through the years and affect breathing and kidney function. He had very limited use of his left hand—just enough to feed himself. As for any other activity, Morty was basically helpless.

But there's a world of difference between helpless and hopeless. Early on, Morty Stein accepted his pain and immobility as a given. Even as a child he chose to get on with the business of living. A special wheelchair made it possible for him to attend school.

That's where I met him. At first, we thought he was a bit weird—you know how kids feel when faced with the unusual or the unknown. We thought he was a freak. But Morty's single-minded passion to get everything he could out of life ultimately touched our hearts. In time, he became everyone's best friend. There wasn't anyone more entertaining, and his spirits were always high. We included him in everything and pushed his wheelchair wherever we went. When the terrain made pushing the chair impossible, we carried him in our arms. Because he didn't make a big deal out of his physical limitations, we forgot he had any. Morty was our inspiration. We were his buddy system.

That relationship continued through high school; even when our careers took us in separate directions, Morty remained an integral part of my life. To be out of touch with him was like being out of touch with part of myself.

After he completed his education, he went on to operate a convalescent hospital, which he ran from his mechanized wheelchair. He moved up and down special ramps from office to office, room to room. I can't imagine a more inspirational example for the patients under his administrative care. Here was a man far more limited than most of them, doing more than many of them had ever done. His very presence had to have a healing effect.

He eventually married a lovely young woman who found him as fascinating as did his friends and co-workers. They had a child, too. Measured by its own standards, Morty's life was a complete success. For him, *nothing* was impossible.

Morty Stein died last year. Scoliosis finally took its toll, and one night his ribs compressed in upon his lungs. His body finally failed him. But as long as Morty lived, he *lived*. And he lives on in my heart today. I know what the words "spirit" and "strength" really mean because of him.

Plato once wrote, "The first and greatest of all man's victories is over self." This has profound implications, because to gain victory over self, one must know what that self is. More than that, we must accept that self with all its failings and foibles. Strength and weakness, we must deal with it all, accept it all. Without that acceptance, there can be no lasting victory.

We're not victims unless we allow ourselves to become victims. We *can* be victors, especially in the battle to recover from physical disability and pain. I've been privileged to see that battle fought and won by thousands of back sufferers. For them to improve took the daily choice to *be*, to *do* and to *have* as much of life's joy as they could grasp. They had a purpose—to get better. To achieve that goal, they took charge of their minds and bodies.

They took charge of their lives. And the lives they created from that moment of choice are monuments of achievement to the human spirit.

At Postural Therapeutics there is a tree. It's not oak, nor redwood. As a matter of fact, it began as a coat rack. Then one day a patient hung his cane up there, deciding he didn't need it anymore. That started a tradition. As patients realized they no longer needed appliances to substitute for self-control, they hung them up on what our staff has come to call the "Orthopedic Appliance Tree." Over the years, that coat rack has expanded to cover one entire wall, decorated with cervical collars, braces, corsets, canes and dozens of other appliances.

Each discard commemorates a minor miracle. A victim became a victor. The only thing more inspiring than to see that tree is to perform that miracle in your own life. Whether you're suffering from back pain or the pain of life it represents, you too can be a victor. Accept responsibility for what you're doing with your life.

Get better.

Index

Page numbers in italic indicate charts or tables.
Page numbers in boldface indicate illustrations.